The Perfect Poison

The Story That Big Food
And Its Friends At The FDA
Don't Want You To Know

Adrienne Samuels, Ph.D.

AS BOOKS

Paperback ISBN: 978-0-9885584-4-1
ebook ISBN: 978-0-9885584-3-4

PRINTED IN THE UNITED STATES OF AMERICA

First Edition: August 1, 2022

Inspired by *The Man Who Sued the FDA*, *It Wasn't Alzheimer's It Was MSG*, and the willingness to think outside the box.

Correspondence should be sent to: Adrienne Samuels, P.O. Box 10028, Chicago, Illinois 60610-0028 USA

Contents

Foreword

Four federal agencies, notably the Food and Drug Administration (FDA), the U.S. Department of Agriculture (USDA), the Environmental Protection Agency (EPA), and the Consumer Products Safety Commission (CPSC) were established at different times when it became apparent that the public needed protection from harm, adulteration and deception.

The objectives of these four federal agencies were commendable. However, regrettably each agency was swiftly diverted from its original purposes, and instead protected the very interests that were creating the problems of harm, adulteration, and deception. These agencies have been infiltrated by industrial interests in a system termed the "revolving door." Individuals from industry are appointed to the agencies, and while serving, weaken or ignore regulations intended to protect consumers. Or, they create new regulations that protect industry's interests rather than protect the public. There are many public servants within these agencies who serve with integrity, and even become whistle blowers, but they are not the administrators who formulate policies and regulations. Upon retirement, these top-echelon return to industry as highly-paid consultants/lobbyists.

For any consumer who suspects that the agency's laxity has affected him/her adversely, it is a long and arduous journey to uncover the truth. Adrienne and her late husband, Jack Samuels are two such consumers. Both suspected that their health was being undermined by a food additive approved officially as safe: monosodium glutamate, a so-called flavor 'enhancer,' added to numerous foods and food products. The Samuels search for the facts was frustrating, torturous, protracted, and filled with confusion and surprises. Ultimately, their search led to understandings and amplifications. The monosodium glutamate enigma was part of a larger issue, encompassing some 3,000 direct food additives, plus some 50,000 indirect additives that have not undergone adequate safety tests; food additives declared to be safe because the manufacturers vouch for their safety without offering proof; tests designed by, and paid for by industry, and manipulated in ways so that the protocols are guaranteed to produce results that show no harm; and input from industry and their legal teams, with little or no representation by independent health professionals or consumers.

What the Samuels uncovered with monosodium glutamate and numerous other substances with glutamic acid in a free state, is applicable to other food additives as well. For example, aspartame (trade name NutraSweet) the synthetic sweetener, has many similar features in its history, testing, and approval of being safe, despite its toxicity.

Regarding food, the FDA's original mandate was to protect consumers from harm, adulteration, and deception. If this original mandate were to be enforced, monosodium glutamate and its related substances, as well as most food additives, could not be permitted in foods. Any food or food product that is made to appear better than it is in reality, would be declared adulterated and deceptive, apart from the more important issue of safety.

Monosodium glutamate, by bestowing a "meaty" flavor, can reduce or replace more costly protein. Thus it is an adulterant and deceptive. Similarly, colors and flavors (both 'natural' and synthetic), added to food to restore what was lost in processing, are adulterants and deceptive because they make the products appear to be of better quality than they are, in reality. Obviously, if foods and food products were seized due to this original mandate, supermarket shelves would be devoid of highly processed foods. What would remain would be whole foods, without questionable additives such as MSG. The results would be better foods, better health, fewer health problems, and reduced medical costs. The MSG issue leads to numerous issues of concern to all.

Beatrice Trum Hunter,
author of *The Mirage of Safety: Food Additives and Federal Policy*

Acknowledgements

This book has been more than thirty years in the writing, with millions of words written on scratch pads and computers before the first manuscript came into being. It grew from knowledge gleaned over the years from people like George Schwartz, John Olney, Russell Blaylock, Jim Turner, Betty Martini, and Maury Silverman who were our eyes and ears from the beginning, and others too numerous to mention, who offered knowledge and support along the way.

Special thanks go to Robert who came to take an oral history from Jack; to Hannah for transcription; Lois, Marlene, Susan, Beatrice, and Ginny, who read early manuscripts and clearly enunciated their shortcomings; Sid who worked with me every step of the way, from changing semicolons to commas and insisting that no statement be made without proof in hand that each statement was true; Marc who found significant errors that no one else had noticed; Bryan who read what I had thought to be a final draft, and made it better; and Colleen on whom I relied to publish the first book that was written. Appreciation goes to Linda Bonvie for her dedication in seeing this updated version to completion, which included her editing help, cover design and layout.

Thanks also go to the good people whose names will not be mentioned for fear they might get slammed, smeared or lose their research grants or positions because they have opposed Big Food or Big Pharma.

Introduction

On November 15, 2011, Jack Samuels suffered a massive heart attack. He died on January 15, 2012 from heart damage exacerbated by complications caused by manufactured free glutamate (MfG) — MfG in the electrode tabs applied to his skin; MfG in the dextrose solution used to deliver the drugs that would crystallize in the non-MfG Ringer's solution; and MfG in the starch, cornstarch, and carrageenan components of the medications given to him when the IVs were withdrawn.

Had the FDA not lied about the toxic potential of MfG, had the medical community not gone along with them, had the MfG in the solutions and meds been identified on product inserts, Jack might be alive today. Had Jack not spent half of the last quarter of his life fibrillating following ingestion of MfG hidden in food, he might not have had the heart attack in the first place.

This book is dedicated to people like Jack with problems that once defied medical diagnosis — people who discovered that elimination of MSG from their diets let them be well.

Clarification of Terms

Sometimes MSG is used as shorthand for the food ingredient monosodium glutamate. At other times it's used to refer to manufactured free glutamate (MfG) — the component in MSG responsible for causing reactions such as fibromyalgia, asthma, migraine headache and heart irregularities like atrial fibrillation.

Confusion arises from the fact that MfG is a component of more than 40 ingredients in addition to monosodium glutamate. And all MfG causes adverse reactions regardless of the names of the ingredients that contain it.

In 1957, when mass production of monosodium glutamate began, adverse reactions to that ingredient began as well. People started realizing that when they ate something with MSG in it, they'd sometimes get lightheaded, have difficulty breathing, get a headache, or some other side effect — all typically called reactions to MSG.

But soon people started noticing those "MSG reactions" could occur when they weren't eating anything that contained MSG.

The cause was actually a component of MSG — manufactured free glutamate, or MfG. Whether strictly accurate or not, consumers continued to call them "MSG reactions."

In this book, the following distinction is made:

MSG: the ingredient called monosodium glutamate.

MfG: manufactured free glutamate, which causes both damage to the arcuate nucleus of the hypothalamus of the brain and detectable reactions such as asthma, skin rash, nausea and vomiting, heart irregularities, seizures, and migraine headaches.

Chapter One

If It Wasn't Alzheimer's...

I don't remember 1989. Not the detail. I just remember it was devastating. For 15 years, Jack had lived with sensitivity to monosodium glutamate. For 15 years, we'd all lived with Jack's sensitivity to monosodium glutamate — but this was something different. This was something new. There were days of fatigue beyond imagination. Sometimes Jack couldn't put a sentence together, and at other times he just lost a critical word or two. Worst of all were the afternoons when Jack couldn't remember what he'd done in the morning.

It wasn't Alzheimer's. Jack's doctor said it wasn't, but how did he know? Did he know Jack's brain didn't have plaques and tangles? He didn't know that. He didn't have a picture of Jack's brain.

The symptoms would come and go, but rarely go. Jack had eliminated monosodium glutamate from his diet. He was very careful. I watched his every move, and I tell you he was very careful. So it wasn't monosodium glutamate, and it wasn't Alzheimer's, because Dr. Levinson said so. But if it wasn't Alzheimer's, then what was it?

In early 1989, Jack had put himself on a diet. Not one of those pound-a-week diets that some people do, but an eat-less-lose-faster-than-you-should diet to meet the needs of someone who found the idea of dieting distasteful and simply wanted to get the job done.

Dull? Unappetizing? Uninspired? This diet would have made anyone ill. He had grapefruit, toast, and cottage cheese for breakfast, a can of tuna fish on Wasa bread for lunch and an insignificant, although at least varied small meal at dinner.

The fat fell away and that was grand, but then something else happened. Two weeks into the diet, Jack lost his ability to speak in whole sentences. There wasn't a thought he could get out without losing a word or two. "Fifty-four years old," Jack said to me, "and I'm falling apart at the seams." Fifty-four years old, Jack was thinking, and I have Alzheimer's disease.

Jack made a tremendous effort to speak slowly and clearly to minimize the appearance of a problem. If you didn't know him well, his halting speech might have seemed quite natural, but if you knew him, you couldn't miss it.

Everyone had a suggestion. Some knew it was stress, "years and years of doing what he did, and doing it well," and all Jack needed was a vacation.

Better yet, he was simply suffering the effects of aging. "Everyone has a little arthritis at 50," (even if the X-rays don't show it). And the memory loss? "Maybe Jack can't remember things as well as he used to, but he still has a better memory than most."

Researcher that I am, I checked out the symptoms of Alzheimer's disease[1] and compared them to Jack's symptoms:

Forgetting recently learned information YES
Difficulty performing familiar tasks YES
Forgetting simple words YES
Getting lost in his own neighborhood YES
Poor or decreased judgment NOT REALLY
Problems with abstract thinking NOT REALLY
Misplacing things YES
Going through rapid mood swings—from calm to anger—for no apparent reason YES
Changes in personality NOT REALLY
Loss of initiative YES

Chapter Two

Then What Was It?

T he title of the book was *In Bad Taste: The MSG Syndrome*[2]. It was written in 1988 by George Schwartz, M.D., a physician who had found that reactions that came after eating food laced with monosodium glutamate would also occur after eating food that contained hydrolyzed vegetable protein, natural flavoring, flavorings, vegetable protein, and/or vegetable, chicken, or beef broth as ingredients.

Dr. Schwartz had been attending a medical convention, grabbing dinner at a Chinese restaurant near his hotel. To hear him tell the story, he'd had no problem with food the first night or the next, but by the end of the week he'd realized he'd become acutely sensitive to monosodium glutamate. How he determined he was also sensitive to hydrolyzed vegetable protein, natural flavoring, flavorings, vegetable protein, and broth we haven't a clue. But he made that determination and shared it with the world. In 1989, our oldest son suggested that his father read *In Bad Taste: The MSG Syndrome*.

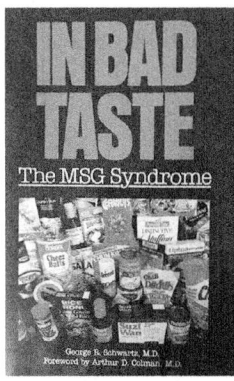

Never mind the book's content. Right on the cover was a picture of the canned tuna Jack had been eating. It's not a big book, and the reading was easy. It took very little time to read it cover to cover.

Jack had long ago eliminated monosodium glutamate from his diet. Now he eliminated all hydrolyzed vegetable protein, natural flavoring, flavorings, vegetable protein, vegetable broth, chicken broth, and beef broth — and the "Alzheimer's" magically disappeared. Gone!

Miraculous? That wasn't the half of it. The general aches and pains, the joint pain that came with age? Disappeared. The chest pain that used to come and go came no more. Frequent trips to the bathroom that had disrupted Jack's sleep at night for at least a year were no longer necessary. Jack suddenly had more energy than he could remember. Moreover, all the recent signs of stress were gone.

Jack wrote to Dr. Schwartz thanking him, and asked some questions. Dr. Schwartz called to respond, and the two men developed an immediate rapport, but Dr. Schwartz couldn't answer all of Jack's questions. Why was Jack sensitive to monosodium glutamate and all the other ingredients that Dr. Schwartz had identified while other people were not? What was it about these products that made Jack ill? Had Dr. Schwartz identified all the products to which Jack would react? What could Jack take or do to prevent having a reaction, and if he did have a reaction, what could he take or do to minimize it?

Who could answer those questions?

Chapter Three

The Search for Understanding

We had questions, lots of questions, and we needed answers. The first, and really the only question we had in 1990, was simple. To what, exactly, was Jack reacting? What was the common element in the monosodium glutamate, hydrolyzed vegetable protein, and the other ingredients named in Dr. Schwartz's book? What foods could I prepare for my husband without producing reactions? Without understanding Jack's sensitivity, there was no way for him to protect himself, and no way for me to help him.

Although I'm a researcher by training, I found it enormously difficult to look for answers to questions when I didn't know what questions to ask. I suspected, but was not really sure, that "monosodium glutamate" would be a good place to start. So, with phone anonymity to cover my embarrassment, I took to the phone book and looked up "dietitian," and "nutrition," and US Food and Drug Administration (FDA). I called colleges and universities. I made phone call after phone call, and when those to whom I spoke couldn't answer my questions, I asked them to tell me who could. If there was such a thing as Google at the time, I knew nothing of it.

I don't remember his name anymore, but someone at the University of Illinois referred me to Dr. Steve Taylor as "the authority on monosodium glutamate." The Institute of Food Technologists (IFT), a trade organization, also referred me to Taylor, who was on the faculty of the University of Nebraska. The American Dietetic Association (ADA), now called the Academy of Nutrition and Dietetics, the American Medical Association (AMA), and the FDA all referred me to The Glutamate Association, the trade organization that represented monosodium glutamate.

I spoke to Richard Cristol at The Glutamate Association. He was warm and caring and assured me that Jack could not possibly be sensitive to monosodium glutamate and he sent me a book that, he said, would prove to me that Jack was not sensitive to monosodium glutamate. He even offered to help me do research that would show that Jack was not sensitive to MSG. Cristol also suggested that I speak to Steve Taylor, who also was warm and caring and assured me that Jack could not be sensitive to monosodium glutamate, and suggested that I speak to Richard Cristol at The Glutamate Association.

It's almost embarrassing to admit, although it did strike me as strange at the time, that these people who did not know Jack or know anything about him, could be so sure it was not MSG causing his problems. And I never challenged them.

I read the book Cristol sent me: *Glutamic Acid: Advances in Biochemistry and Physiology*[3]. It contained the proceedings of a symposium held in May 1978 in Milan, Italy, for what seemed to be the thinly veiled purpose of appearing to prove that monosodium glutamate was safe. I knew that a significant number of studies done by independent researchers (and not mentioned in the book) had demonstrated that monosodium glutamate had toxic potential[4]. But, with a single exception[5], researchers contributing to the book (who were supported, at least in part, by the glutamate industry) found monosodium glutamate to be harmless[6,7]. I still can't believe that it never occurred to me that the symposium and the book were simply designed to convince people like me that monosodium glutamate was a harmless food additive. It never occurred to me that authors and editors were being paid by the U.S. manufacturer of monosodium glutamate to convince the public that monosodium glutamate was "safe."

My husband had a potentially life-threatening malady, and by endorsing the badly flawed studies reproduced in this book, editors Lloyd J. Filer, Jr., Silvio Garattini, Morley R. Kare, W. Ann Reynolds, and Richard J. Wurtman were digging Jack's grave. Only later did I begin to entertain the thought that Andrew Ebert, chairman of the International Glutamate Technical Committee (IGTC), would be acting as undertaker[8].

It didn't take a whole lot of brain power, just a bit of carefully focused attention and a yearning for the truth to realize that the research reported was, for the most part, built on inappropriate methodology and/or drew conclusions that didn't follow from study results. There was, however, one paper by John Olney, M.D.[5] that appeared to be based on well-done research, and I set out to read more. I was focused. I wasn't interested in inadequate researchers. I needed to find out what Jack was reacting to.

I searched the Index Medicus and read it all. When I couldn't understand what an author was saying, I went to the children's section of the library and took out elementary science books. I consulted dictionaries, encyclopedias, books and journals. Although some of the scientific details were beyond my immediate comprehension, being an experimental psychologist by training, I had no difficulty "reading" the scientific method. Clearly, there were two types of studies: those that set out to uncover the truth, whatever that might be[4], and those that set out to lend credibility to the notion that monosodium glutamate was safe[6,7].

I was reading constantly, almost voraciously, without finding answers to my questions. I'd discovered that some studies seemed to conclude that monosodium glutamate was a harmless substance, while others concluded that monosodium glutamate was toxic. That was very interesting to Adrienne the researcher, but told me nothing about the nature of the ingredients that caused Jack's debilitating reactions. And that was what I was desperate to know.

The answers to my questions did come eventually, not from studies of the safety/toxicity of monosodium glutamate, but from individual consumers, manufacturers, food chemists, food technologists, food encyclopedias, trade magazines, people Jack met on airplanes, and above all, intuition. From those sources, we came to realize that all the adverse reaction triggers named by Dr. Schwartz contained free glutamic acid, i.e., glutamic acid that existed without being bound in protein. Then, as consumers began reporting that they reacted to products in addition to those with ingredients named by Dr. Schwartz, we began to appreciate the fact that their reactions were always associated with ingredients that contained manufactured free glutamic acid, be it separated from protein through some manufacturing process or through fermentation, or be it produced by genetically engineered bacteria grown to secrete monosodium glutamate through their cell walls.

From trade journal articles and advertisements written in the early 1990s, we learned that ingredients containing manufactured free glutamic acid could be substituted for monosodium glutamate without sacrificing the perception of enhanced taste that MSG is famous for. From trade journal articles, we also learned that people in the flavoring industry understood there was profit to be made from monosodium glutamate substitutes, ingredients that when included on food ingredient labels would give no indication that there was any manufactured free glutamic acid in their products[9-11]. Industry calls these "clean labels."

From a 1994 study done by Kimber Rundlett and Daniel Armstrong[12], we learned that processed food containing free L-glutamic acid invariably contains free D-glutamic acid. With that knowledge, we were able to search out information about the various impurities found in monosodium glutamate and the other ingredients that contained manufactured/processed free glutamic acid. We even found a 1977 account of the impurities present in monosodium glutamate tucked away in the files of the FDA's Dockets Management office[13]. Thus, it became clear that the free glutamic acid component of monosodium glutamate, which was manufactured and contained impurities, was not identical to the glutamic acid component of unadulterated protein in plants, fruits, grains, meat, vegetables, and the human body.

In time we found that Ajinomoto Co., Inc. had become the sole producer of MSG in the United States, and much more. From the Ajinomoto Group Global Website, we learned:

- That it commands a dominant share of the global amino acids market in food, feed, pharmaceutical, and other segments.

- That the fact that it has the advanced production technology and capacity to ensure stable supply of amino acid-based products is the core of its competitive strength.

- That it produces nearly 20 amino acids at 27 locations around the world with a global production system comprising a network of strategically-located plants, reliable supplies of optimum materials and microbes, and state-of-the-art processes.

- As a leader in what it calls "umami science" (information and research), Ajinomoto Co., Inc. supports various organizations that provide what we call "brain-washing" about umami. Examples of those associations include the Umami Information Center, The Glutamate Association, the International Glutamate Information Service, and the International Glutamate Technical Committee.

On the Internet, we found copies of patents associated with the production of monosodium glutamate[14]. From those patents, we learned that beginning in 1957, Ajinomoto's monosodium glutamate was being made by a process of bacterial fermentation wherein carefully selected genetically modified bacteria fed on various carbohydrate media secreted glutamic acid through their cell walls — a fact that was later confirmed by a 1996 article we found in the *Encyclopedia of Common Natural Ingredients Used in Food, Drugs, and Cosmetics*[15].

We also learned that the information in Ajinomoto's patents bore little resemblance to the descriptions of monosodium glutamate production found on the website of The Glutamate Association. According to The Glutamate Association:

"[Monosodium glutamate] is usually produced through fermentation, a process similar to that used in making beer, vinegar and yogurt. The process usually begins with the fermentation of corn, sugar beets or sugar cane"[16], or "[Monosodium glutamate] is produced by fermentation, a process similar to that used in making beer, vinegar and yogurt. Carbohydrates from crops such as corn, sugar beets/cane or cassava are fermented to produce glutamate which is purified and crystallized before drying"[17].

In contrast, according to Ajinomoto's patents, monosodium glutamate was being produced using bacterial fermentation, a process whereby carefully selected genetically modified bacteria secrete free glutamic acid through their cell walls[14].

Was I so focused on finding the key to Jack's sensitivity to MSG that I saw, but didn't notice, that the studies that proclaimed the safety of

MSG were actually flawed — flawed, I would later say, to the point of being fraudulent.

Little did I know that what I then considered to be meaningless discrepancies were more akin to scientific fraud.

Chapter Four

A Decade Like No Other

With the advent of *In Bad Taste: The MSG Syndrome*, a whole new world opened up. It was 1989, the Alzheimer's was gone, and Jack knew not to get into anything that George Schwartz had mentioned in his book. Jack's reactions to monosodium glutamate were as before: monosodium glutamate alone caused mood swings and fatigue, while monosodium glutamate in combination with alcohol brought on anaphylactic shock. The greatest difference lay in the fact that Jack now realized that his reactions were precipitated by all kinds of ingredients that contained manufactured free glutamic acid — not just the one ingredient called monosodium glutamate. Confusing as it was at the time, and as it continues to be, those who are sensitive to the manufactured free glutamic acid (MfG) found in monosodium glutamate and many other ingredients, began to refer to all ingredients that contain MfG as MSG.

Armed with the knowledge that there was MfG (which at the time we still referred to as "MSG") hidden in processed food, and the awareness that Jack dared not drink anything alcoholic outside of our own home, his health was far better than it had been in years. Life was tolerable and he was content to tolerate it.

I had taken Jack's sensitivity to MSG more seriously than he had, and in 1989, when I read that the FDA and the U.S. Department of Agriculture (USDA) were taking public testimony relevant to the National Labeling and Education Act of 1990 (NLEA), I insisted that Jack find out if he could attend and give testimony regarding the toxic potential of MSG. Jack knew there was no point to it, and told me so. "What for? Why should I bother? It will be a waste of time. Besides, I don't have the time."

THE NLEA HEARINGS

When Jack called the FDA office in Chicago to ask if he could give testimony, the person he spoke to seemed genuinely excited by the prospect of having someone talk about MSG. She asked that by nine the next morning, he give her names of three people he'd bring with him. With less than 24 hours to identify MSG-sensitive people in Chicago, Jack called Dr. Schwartz, who was pleased to come from New Mexico to testify. Then Jack called and confirmed two Chicago people whose names Dr. Schwartz had given him.

The series of NLEA hearings began Monday, October 16, 1989 in Chicago. Speakers focused on the general issue of nutrition label content. Participants generally agreed that nutrition labeling should be mandatory and nutrition labels should include cholesterol and fat content, with fats divided into saturated and unsaturated (or monounsaturated and polyunsaturated). Consumers stressed the need for serving sizes to be more uniform and suggested using common household measures, such as a cup or tablespoon.

Industry, we learned, had a different agenda. A representative from Company One testified to the need to have fat content spelled out in milligrams. A representative from Company Two testified to the need to have fat content listed per serving. Actually, each was asking to have fat content listed in a way that would leave consumers thinking they were getting less fat than they actually were.

Before the Chicago meeting, we believed the NLEA hearings were being called to work out the details of labeling that would best provide consumers with information about the food they might buy. When we left the meeting, we understood that the meeting had been called for the benefit of the food industry, whose sales, translated into profit, were the only concern. It wasn't until sometime later that we learned just how far some of these giants of industry would go to turn a dollar and to what extremes the FDA would go to back them.

WASHINGTON

It was during the NLEA hearing that Dr. Schwartz was invited to Washington by the FDA to begin a dialogue on the safety of monosodium glutamate. That meeting would be an important step toward clear and full labeling of the MSG in processed foods – labeling that would alert Jack to the presence of MSG and allow him to lead a normal life.

On the day before he was scheduled to leave for Washington, however, Dr. Schwartz called to say he'd received a Federal Express letter from the FDA, contending his beliefs about MSG were unfounded, and his Washington trip would be a waste of time.

There was no question about it; Dr. Schwartz was cancelling his trip. He was adamant. He knew it would be nothing more than a waste of time and money. Jack, on the other hand, saw an opportunity that might never come again. In the end, Dr. Schwartz went to Washington and Jack accompanied him for moral support.

Jack couldn't wait to call me after the meeting with news of how it went:

> "We've done it! I wish you had been with us. It was incredible.
>
> "There were 10 people from the FDA. Very reserved. Very cold when we came in, but they listened to us. They listened to what we had to say. Clearly, when we left in the late afternoon, we knew they cared.
>
> "Young was there. Commissioner Young. FDA Commissioner Frank E. Young. He couldn't stay the whole time, but when he left, he told the others they must take careful note of what we said because there was a problem here and it had to be remedied.
>
> "Honey, I wish you had been with us. They just didn't understand. And now that they understand, it won't be long before all manufactured glutamic acid will be identified on food labels, and you won't have to worry ever again about me dying from hidden MSG.
>
> "Not everyone saw things our way, you understand. A man named Ronk, in particular, actually looked evil. I

could just see him making mental notes as though he was trying to send them by telepathy to The Glutamate Association. I wonder how long it will be before the 'Glutes'[A] find out about our meeting. I wonder if it will be Ronk who tells them, or maybe Glinsmann. I wonder if one or the other is on their payroll. But that's something we'll probably never know. And it doesn't matter, honey, because now that they know there really is a problem, they'll do something about it. Honey, I wish you could have been there."

But in short order, Jack's excitement turned to skepticism. Days turned into weeks, and copies of the minutes of his meeting promised by the FDA failed to materialize. When at last they did arrive, the only resemblance to the meeting that Dr. Schwartz and Jack had attended was in the names of the people who had been there.

Jack was frustrated. He simply didn't understand how the FDA, the agency charged with overseeing the health and welfare of consumers[18], could take on the demeanor of a chameleon. When Jack and Dr. Schwartz left the meeting in December 1989, Jack believed that because the FDA now understood the problems MSG-sensitive people were facing, something would be done to remedy the situation. Jack wasn't sure about Dr. Schwartz, but after receiving those minutes, Jack was faced with contemplating the possibility that the FDA might not be the honorable agency he thought it to be. In 1989, that was something he was not willing to consider.

PICKING UP SPEED

By the time 1990 came, we were picking up speed gathering information. I was reading the medical literature to understand adverse reactions, researching to find answers. Jack was focused on finding opportunities to educate anyone in a position to effect change.

What was causing Jack's reactions? By January 1990, we realized that what we were calling monosodium glutamate would always be found in hydrolyzed vegetable protein, hydrolyzed plant protein, autolyzed yeast, hydrolyzed milk protein, sodium caseinate, calcium caseinate, and anything else that was hydrolyzed.[B] We had yet to learn that it's not the ingredient called "monosodium glutamate" that caused his reactions, but its free glutamic acid component, MfG. We also had good reason to suspect that this MfG would be found, at least some of the time, in ingredients called natural flavors, natural flavoring, malt flavoring, high flavored yeast, flavoring, broth, yeast extract, yeast nutrients, and seasoning.

In addition to finding hydrolysis-processed MfG in a variety of processed soups, sauces, salad dressing, sausages, processed meats, frozen dinners, and pizza, we found it in cookies, breakfast cereal, mineral supplements, bread, and cocoa mix. We'd been told, but hadn't verified the information, that hydrolysis-processed MfG could also be found in dairy products. And we'd been told that natural flavoring included in meat products often contained a hydrolyzed protein product made from pork, which was being used in processed poultry and beef products without being identified as pork.

Much of what we learned came from books, newspapers, magazines and journals. Some things came to us through people who volunteered information. To find other things, we traveled.

SAN FRANCISCO

On Thursday, February 8, 1990, Jack flew to San Francisco to testify before a committee of the Board of Supervisors of the City and County of San Francisco. He'd been invited by Supervisor Wendy Nelder, who, with Supervisor Angela Alioto, had drafted an ordinance requiring San Francisco restaurants to disclose the presence of MSG on their menus. Nelder and Alioto were presenting that proposed ordinance to a committee of the San Francisco Board of Supervisors[19].

On the appointed day, Jack met briefly with Nelder, who asked him to visit the others before whom he would testify. All, however, were too busy to see him. When he later entered the room where the ordinance was to be considered, the cold silence emanating from those super-busy people bordered on hostility. It was clear that no ordinance would be approved that afternoon.

As a scheduled speaker, Jack made a brief statement in support of the ordinance. Then, from the audience, Steve Taylor rose to inform the group that he just happened to be in San Francisco, and had read that an ordinance to require the labeling of MSG on restaurant menus was being considered. Taylor explained that he felt obligated to come to the meeting and inform the commissioners that they would be making a terrible mistake in labeling MSG because he knew it was absolutely safe.

Jack found it interesting that Taylor forgot to tell the Supervisors he was on the payroll of The Glutamate Association and/or the IGTC[8]. I still wonder how much Taylor got paid for "just happening to be in town," and whether it was The Glutamate Association, the IGTC, or Ajinomoto directly that paid him.

If Jack had thought about it at the time, he might have noticed that there was great similarity between San Francisco and what he and Dr. Schwartz had experienced in Washington a month earlier. The settings were different, but the involvement of the glutamate industry had been the same. In San Francisco, he saw the Glutes represented by Steve Taylor. In Washington, the Glutes were apparently represented by some person or persons at the FDA. In both cases, any material presented by MSG-sensitive people would be ignored. There'd be no discussion of the toxic potential of MSG.

CHICAGO NOMSG

On June 18, 1990, Jack and I hosted the first Chicago area meeting of the National Organization Mobilized to Stop Glutamate (NOMSG), a group formed by people who had read George Schwartz' book. On June 20, we held a NOMSG meeting at the Skokie Public Library. On June 21, Jack made a presentation before his Kiwanis Club. In all cases, the turnouts were modest.

On September 5, we flew to Washington, where I testified before the Advisory Committee of the Food and Drug Administration.

THE AMA

Sometime in early 1990, Jack had become aware that a board member of a hospital he was serving as administrator also sat on the board of the American Medical Association (AMA), an organization he was most interested in approaching. Not being shy, he'd asked for an introduction, hoping the AMA would allow him to formally request its assistance in having MSG labeled. Where once he'd been reluctant to pursue appropriate labeling of MSG, now he was determined that MSG should be identified when used in processed foods.

His meeting was held on September 26, 1990 with an 8-10-member special committee comprised of AMA executives. The committee members were extremely rude, and when the relatively short meeting ended, all but one quickly left the room. The remaining gentleman apologized for the manner in which Jack had been treated. He told Jack that two years earlier, William Crook, M.D., a pediatric allergist, had appeared before the same group asking the AMA to endorse his finding that candida had become a major medical problem. The AMA member went on to say that Dr. Crook had been treated as rudely as Jack had, even though Cook wasn't as strident in his presentation. He then reported that although not well received by the AMA, Crook had gone on with his work, and now candida was accepted as a legitimate medical diagnosis. The AMA member suggested that Jack keep up his work on MSG, and perhaps the outcome would be the same for him as it had been for Dr. Crook.

Jack reflected on what this doctor had told him. It occurred to him that the difference between Crook's case and his own case might lie in the fact that in Jack's case there was a rich and powerful industry determined not to lose the cash cow it had in flavor enhancers, even while knowing that MSG was harmful.

Jack wasn't the only one to approach the AMA. In 1991, the AMA passed a resolution submitted by its Michigan chapter calling for the organization to encourage the FDA to "...mandate labeling of all foods containing even small amounts of additive L-glutamic acid so that individuals wanting to avoid this substance may do so"[20]. How it sneaked past the glutamate industry observers we'll never know, but they remedied the situation in 1992 when the AMA Council on Scientific Affairs recommended:

> "...that until such time as L-glutamic acid in any form has been shown to pose a significant public health hazard, or until biological non-equivalence of monosodium glutamate and L-glutamate has been demonstrated, the AMA should not advise the FDA to mandate the labeling of all foods containing added L-glutamic acid"[21].

WASHINGTON AND CBN

On October 21, we returned to Washington and spent seven days during which we visited attorney Jim Turner (Dr. Olney's lawyer and one of the original Nader's Raiders), who shared documentation of the MSG "controversy" dating back to 1969. Gailon Totheroh and his television crew from the Christian Broadcasting Network (CBN) interviewed us. We visited friends who might have friends in high places. We stayed at the Residence Inn in Bethesda, where we had a full kitchen and Jack could cook our meals.

At the time, Totheroh worked for Pat Robertson at CBN News. A few years earlier, Robertson had done a segment on the dangers of aspartame, reporting that he'd begun to have difficulty speaking, pulling words and connecting thoughts. Then, with the help of his personal physician, and after extensive testing, someone had recalled that Robertson had recently begun drinking diet soda that contained aspartame.

We heard this story from a friend who'd seen Robertson's first program on the hazards of using aspartame. The following day, Jack called the 700 Club, Robertson's TV newsmagazine, and explained to Totheroh that if Robertson was reacting to aspartame, he'd also likely be sensitive to MSG. Six months later, Jack received a call from Totheroh indicating he was ready to do a segment on MSG. The interview that took place in Washington was the first of a number of segments that Totheroh did for the 700 Club on the dangers of MSG.

NOHA

Toward the end of the year, we attended our first meeting of the Nutrition for Optimal Health Association (NOHA), an organization dedicated to educating people on the health benefits of sound nutrition. It was at a NOHA lecture that we first met Beatrice Trum Hunter, the author of many outstanding books on health issues, and former food editor for *Consumers' Research*. I'd hazard to say that there was no person more knowledgeable on health issues than Hunter, no person with more integrity, and no person more pleased to share her knowledge with others. We've been proud to call her colleague and friend.

JOHN OLNEY

On Friday, December 28, we visited Drs. John Olney and Madelon Price at Washington University in St. Louis. I had questions about the animal research Olney had conducted in 1969 and the 1970s[22], and the badly flawed industry-sponsored studies with which the glutamate industry had challenged his findings[6]. Price was a colleague of Olney, and had worked with him on a number of studies.

We came away from that meeting with a far better understanding of what the research climate had been during the 1970s, and with tremendous respect for Dr. Olney, a brilliant researcher who'd put his career at risk by standing up to the glutamate industry.

AFTER SO MUCH RESEARCH, WHAT HAD I LEARNED?

As we moved from meeting to meeting and from place to place, we were gathering information. Jack was actively soliciting help from people who might help us understand the nature of MSG, and I was reading everything I could find on the subject.

I must have spent most of 1990 in the library. By January 1991, I'd read everything I could find that might be remotely related to MSG. I'd labored through card catalogs in rooms without air conditioning, and then turned to the Index Medicus bound in unwieldy tomes to unearth the secrets of the glutamate industry.

When everything was put together, what had I found?

I'd come to realize that any glutamic acid ingested as a single amino acid would cause MSG reactions in people who exceeded their tolerances for the substance. I'd also come to understand that MfG could be intentionally produced/manufactured in food or chemical plants by acid hydrolysis, autolysis, enzymolysis, or bacterial fermentation, and that MfG would be produced, possibly unintentionally, when a protein source was left to ferment. I found that MfG can be produced through a complex cooking process wherein a product referred to as a "reaction flavor" is produced from a combination of specific amino acids, reducing sugars, animal or vegetable fats or oils, and optional ingredients including hydrolyzed vegetable protein[23]. It was only later that I would learn that acid-hydrolyzed proteins contain carcinogenic mono and dichloro propanols[24], and later yet that reaction flavors contain carcinogenic heterocyclic amines[25].

And all that information stood in sharp contrast to the flood of literature from the glutamate industry assuring the public as well as health care professionals that MSG was a harmless food additive. Yet, it still didn't penetrate my consciousness that the American public was purposely being deceived so a large Japanese company could line its pockets with gold.

THEY CALL THEM DISCREPANCIES

As pieces of the puzzle began to come together, we began to give serious consideration to the discrepancies in the published literature, the so-called scientific studies. We knew from personal experience as well as from reports of others that adverse reactions such as asthma, heart irregularities, and migraine headaches could be caused by MfG. We also knew from well-done published studies that MfG kills brain cells, disrupts the endocrine system, and causes retinal degeneration[22]. How could it be, then, that the glutamate industry was able to produce studies from which it could conclude that MSG was safe?

Animal studies were easy to understand. John Olney had told us how the Glutes produced studies they claimed were failed attempted replications, with procedures different enough to guarantee that toxic doses had not been administered, or that all evidence that nerve cells had died would have been obscured. Criticisms of those animal studies had been published, but the key to understanding human studies eluded us.

In the privacy of our kitchen, Jack and I hashed and rehashed one study after another, trying to understand how data could be manipulated to come up with the predetermined conclusion that monosodium glutamate could be considered a harmless flavor enhancer. We could see that each of their studies produced negative results (there was no difference between the reactions of people who'd ingested monosodium glutamate and those who hadn't) — which was interesting, but proved nothing about the safety of monosodium glutamate.

Finding no difference between two groups doesn't **prove** there's no difference between them. The following examples illustrate the reasoning.

Example 1: Suppose it's known unequivocally from space missions that there's life on Mars, and all Martians (group 1) have two heads. One day, an alien spacecraft lands in your backyard, and several aliens emerge (group 2). If the visiting aliens had three heads, we'd know they weren't from Mars, and there must be life on other planets. (There's clearly a difference between the two groups of aliens.) However, if the visiting aliens had two heads (just like the Martians), they might be from Mars, or they might come from another planet. Perhaps there are two-headed aliens on another planet.

Example 2: Suppose that subjects are given purple dye number 12 or a placebo, and the number of headaches reported by each group is the same. If reports of headaches had been significantly greater in the group given purple dye, we could have concluded, with a certain amount of confidence, that purple dye caused headaches. However, since reports of headaches were approximately the same for both groups, we wouldn't know what to conclude. It might be that purple dye doesn't cause headaches. It might be that subjects were eating something with purple dye in it during the studies, giving the placebo group headaches, or that purple dye only causes headaches in females and all the subjects were males.

Drawing conclusions based on failure to find a difference is grossly inappropriate[26-28]. Given the statistical model used in the glutamate industry studies, rigorous demonstration of the truth of the null hypothesis (that there's no difference between groups) is a logical impossibility[26].

Failure to find a statistically significant difference between groups may provide useful information for planning your next experiment, but it proves nothing. If you find something, then you find it. If you don't find something, it might be because it's hiding, because you didn't look in the right place, because you're inept, or because someone paid you not to find it. Yet, the glutamate industry people have used these negative studies as a basis for asserting that monosodium glutamate should be considered a harmless flavor enhancer. But that's not the disturbing part of the story. What's disturbing is that the "scientists" at the FDA charged with our well-being, chose and still choose, not to notice.

Through careful reading of these studies[7], I had become aware that none met the assumptions of the statistics used and cited, so conclusions drawn from each and every study were invalid.

But there was something more. In the double-blind studies, where subjects ingested monosodium glutamate on one occasion and a placebo on another, researchers reported that there were as many responses to placebos as there were to monosodium glutamate test material. And that, we knew, could not be true. Unless, of course, those placebos were not truly inert, as placebos must be.[C] But that was unthinkable. It was unthinkable that anyone — anyone — would lace placebos with material that might cause adverse reactions.

QUESTIONING THE UNTHINKABLE

By the beginning of 1991, however, we were thinking the unthinkable.

Jack had signed up to give testimony in Washington, DC before the FASEB (Federation of American Societies for Experimental Biology) hearing on the Safety of Amino Acids Used in Dietary Supplements. The open meeting, required by law, was held for public input into the safety of amino acids in dietary supplements, which was being debated by the FDA following the L-tryptophan debacle when more than 35 people died and over 100 became disabled following ingestion of L-tryptophan sold as a dietary supplement. We had been fairly certain it would be L-tryptophan that would take the center stage, but on the chance that he'd be able to give input on the toxicity of manufactured free glutamic acid (MfG), Jack decided to make the trip. So it was that Jack stood up at that meeting and suggested there was something wrong with the glutamate industry placebos used in studies of the safety of MSG, leading to the loud protestations of IGTC Chairman Ebert and the eventual disclosure of the fact that the IGTC had been lacing the placebos supplied to IGTC researchers with neurotoxic, endocrine-disrupting, adverse-reaction-causing aspartame.

(Actually, Ebert didn't mention that aspartame was "neurotoxic, endocrine disrupting, and adverse reaction causing." I just added that because it's true.)

It wasn't quite a shot in the dark, but it certainly was a long-shot — and Jack won the prize, for there was Ebert on his feet, protesting that the glutamate industry's integrity was being impugned.

The long-shot paid off immediately, although we didn't know it for another two years. In a letter dated February 6, 1991, Sue Anne Anderson, Senior Staff Scientist with the Life Sciences Research Office at FASEB asked Ebert for information about the vehicles used for administration of monosodium glutamate and placebos in IGTC-sponsored double-blind studies. In response, a March 22, 1991 letter to Anderson from the IGTC chairman stated that "since the completion of the work described in [1978], the sample has been modified to replace the sucrose with the low-calorie sweetener aspartame in both the placebo and sample with MSG"[29].

Translated for those who might not immediately understand the importance of what was being said, Ebert admitted that since 1978, all the placebos in double-blind IGTC-sponsored studies had contained aspartame — an ingredient that causes brain lesions, endocrine disorders, migraine headache, depression and all the other adverse reactions that can be caused by the MfG found in monosodium glutamate, hydrolyzed protein products, autolyzed yeast, etc.[30-31].

Today, we know that all of the industry-sponsored studies were of similar design, created by, or with the cooperation of IGTC chairman Ebert; that the details varied only slightly; that all failed to meet the requirements of the statistical models on which their conclusions were based, and all used aspartame in placebos[7], leading us to conclude that taken as a whole, the glutamate industry studies bordered on, or were flawed to the point of, being fraudulent.[D]

THE PAYOFF

It was 1993 before we discovered that Ebert had responded to Anderson, admitting that the placebos in the IGTC-sponsored studies contained aspartame. We were in Washington, DC, to testify before the FASEB Expert Panel taking testimony on the safety of monosodium glutamate in food when I became aware, for the first time, that there was a law stating that all communications with the FDA be filed in dockets housed at the Docket Management Office in Rockville, Md. But not until the day before we were scheduled to leave Washington did it occur to me that I needed to read all dockets pertaining to MSG. It was nearly Dockets closing time on that last scheduled day in Washington, and Jack was badgering me to finish and leave — which I refused to do. Instead,

I passed Jack a number of folders and asked him to go through them in the hope that he might find something, but more for the sake of keeping him quiet.

"My name! Here's my name!"

Jack saw his name in a copy of testimony given February 4, 1991 by Andrew Ebert on the "Evaluation of Amino Acids and Related Products"[32]. We'd previously seen a copy of that testimony, and had found nothing noteworthy in it, but as Jack looked through Ebert's testimony and read from documents in the docket that followed it, he found Ebert's letter to Anderson stating that the placebos being used by IGTC researchers contained aspartame[29].

Poor Andrew Ebert. Betrayed by the FDA's recordkeeping system. We can only guess that in replying to Anderson, Ebert had no way of knowing what we knew about the composition of his placebos, and didn't dare lie. In fact, while the statements of the glutamate industry are often deceptive and misleading, I don't remember seeing more than one out-and-out lie. They have been known to fail to answer questions, and to respond to question with irrelevant answers, yet to my knowledge, have never been challenged by the FDA, USDA, or EPA. The fact that Ebert responded to Anderson, and actually answered her question, is intriguing. Even more interesting is the fact that Anderson asked the question in the first place.

It appears to be Glute policy to avoid **saying** anything that might be contested, it being relatively easy for a critic to contest words whether spoken or written, while being difficult to dispute something that hasn't been said. I've only recently noticed that when the truth about the toxicity of MSG or MfG is the subject, the FDA does the same thing – ignoring a petition to remove MSG and MfG from the GRAS list, for example.

INDUSTRY'S FDA?

As you might imagine, Jack brought the information to the attention of both FASEB and the FDA. We were still naïve enough to believe that the FDA might consider the fact that there were studies clearly demonstrating that MSG causes brain lesions, endocrine disorders, migraine headaches, seizures, irritable bowel, heart irregularities, depression and more, while all the studies submitted to the FDA as evidence of the safety of MSG, when reviewed in their entirety, had to be considered fraudulent. That's what we believed. We were naïve.

We'd started our quest with one question: "What is the nature of the products that cause Jack's reactions?" Before we found the answer to that question, we'd found the very disturbing answer to a question we'd not even considered. Given that there's incontrovertible evidence that MSG has toxic potential, how could the glutamate industry produce human studies from which it could conclude MSG was safe?

The answer? Guarantee the results by lacing placebos in double-blind studies with aspartame, an excitotoxic amino acid known to cause not only brain damage, but adverse reactions identical to those caused by the excitotoxic glutamic acid in MSG.

We're from Chicago, and we've heard it said more than once that public officials can be bought. We'd heard you could get a highway contract with the city or state if you knew the right people, and you could get a building permit without waiting if you had the right connections. We had no reason to doubt that, but neither Jack nor I had ever considered there might be people so filled with greed that they would harm and even kill their own family and friends for profit.

We'd been at a disadvantage. Detectives will tell you that to track perpetrators you have to think like a perpetrator. You have to get inside their heads to catch them, and we'd had no practice. In 1993, however, we began to play catch-up. It had become abundantly clear that, in the words of novelist Michael Crichton, "business is war"[33], and we knew for certain that if the glutamate industry was being run as a war, then both it and their FDA colleagues were enemy combatants.

It wasn't until years later that it became clear to us that much of corporate American was involved in intentionally feeding toxic, endocrine-disrupting, adverse reaction-causing manufactured amino acids to every American, including the unborn. We didn't yet know enough to suspect that the FDA might be little more than a front for both the pharmaceutical and food industries, dumbing down consumers with toxic food and pharmaceuticals sanctioned and made possible by the people you and I had elected to public office.

Dr. Schwartz and Jack had been to Washington. They'd seen the FDA in action on behalf of the glutamate industry. I had reviewed the literature and found there was nothing to suggest that MSG is safe. We didn't yet understand the FDA/industry partnership — neither the fact that there was such a partnership nor how well developed and deep rooted it was. But we knew we were looking at something more ominous than sloppy research.

In 1991, we picked up chatter about a new study to be commissioned by the FDA on the safety of monosodium glutamate. There was some talk at the time of hiring someone other than FASEB to do the study, but it didn't happen. It crossed my mind that a different organization might fail to come up with the "right" conclusions, and that made FASEB the FDA's ultimate choice. FASEB had never found anything wrong with any food substance studied for the FDA, not even trans fatty acids[34].

THE GLUTAMATE INDUSTRY IN ACTION

In 1990–91, there was an eruption of glutamate industry literature/propaganda aimed at health-conscious people. The Glutes know what they're doing, and they hire professionals to accomplish their goals. The most notable professional organization at the time was the International Food Information Council (IFIC), which represents itself as an "independent" organization, and sends attractive brochures to dietitians, nutritionists, hospitals, schools, the media, and politicians proclaiming the safety of monosodium glutamate among other things. An IFIC "Communication Plan" dated July-December 1991 detailed methods for scuttling a *60 Minutes* program on MSG that was in the works, or, failing that, provided for crisis management[35].

But there's more. Much more. The Glutes have given generous donations to influential bodies such as the American Dietetic Association[36]. We've found glutamate industry material in the Mayo Clinic Nutrition Letter[37], the University of California Berkeley Wellness Letter[38-39], and material published by the American Association of Retired People (AARP)[40].

We'd seen their propaganda in newspapers and popular magazines, too, including *The Oregonian*, *Better Homes and Gardens*, *Women's Day*, and *Family Circle*. Each time one of these articles came to our attention, one of us wrote to the author or the editor who couldn't have cared less.

Although it appeared to us that the Glutes had Washington sewed up, they were clearly nervous. They have a history of turning out studies and mass-producing propaganda whenever the integrity of monosodium glutamate is threatened, and that's what they were doing. We thought the activity might have stemmed from the fact that we'd sent the FDA a copy of my review of the literature[41] and the FDA was calling for a study of the "safety" of MSG to counteract it. But my review wasn't printed until January 1991, so it couldn't have been that.

The Glutes were certainly aware that Jack and I were asking questions — questions about MSG and questions about their research, because we often addressed those questions directly to them. Possibly more worrisome for them had been the 1988 publication of *In Bad Taste: The MSG Syndrome*, and the formation of the new consumer group, NOMSG. In 1990, the glutamate industry had no way of being sure what was on NOMSG's agenda.

It wasn't until sometime later that we began to understand the structure and function of the glutamate industry's propaganda/crisis-management system. One of their stock strategies for drawing attention to themselves and the safety of monosodium glutamate is to set up workshops, symposia, and meetings where they extol the virtues of monosodium glutamate — and then send press releases to those who take paid advertising from The Glutamate Association, the IGTC, or one of their member food or drug companies[42]. They also publish the papers that come from their workshops, etc. in supplement sections of industry-friendly journals that accept such papers without peer review[43]. Few readers will make a distinction between articles that come through the peer-review process and those that don't.

In August 1991, for example, the Glutes held an MSG workshop organized by their longtime researcher and spokesperson, L. J. Filer Jr., M.D., Ph.D., who was then emeritus professor of pediatrics at the University of Iowa College of Medicine in Iowa City[8]. Predictably, presenters included IGTC researchers and spokespersons Susan Schiffman, Ph.D., L.D. Stegink, Ph.D., Steve Taylor, Ph.D., and John Fernstrom, Ph.D., all of whom were referred to as a "group of experts representing a variety of disciplines." We knew them to be representatives of a variety of disciplines reclining under the umbrella of the IGTC[8].

60 MINUTES

In early 1990, we'd become aware that a *60 Minutes* segment on MSG was in the works, and over the course of its development, Jack provided information to producers Grace Dickhaus and Roz Karson, and a "heads-up" to the *Wall Street Journal*.

In March 1991, a producer for the CBS news show had called Ajinomoto announcing that they were thinking of doing a segment on monosodium glutamate. According to the *Wall Street Journal* a group of trade associations thereupon launched one of the largest pre-emptive campaigns in public relations history. According to the *Wall Street Journal*, "A crisis-management team specializing in *60 Minutes* damage control has been hired to help the glutamate industry execute an elaborate game plan to forestall a repeat of the 1989 Alar-on-apples scare"[44]. It was a copy of that crisis management team's "July-December 1991 Communications Plan"[35] designed (or possibly simply distributed) by the IFIC that Jack had sent to the *Wall Street Journal*. We'd received the "war plan" for IFIC's assault on *60 Minutes* from an anonymous source on September 4, 1991.

Prior to the advent of the *60 Minutes* feature, I had developed relationships with food editors from most of the major newspapers. From time to time, one of them carried a story about MSG that included a mention of consumer concerns. In 1991, I circulated my report, "MSG: A Review of the Literature and Critique of Industry Sponsored Research"[41] sending a copy to the FDA. An article, "Monosodium Glutamate: Food for Thought but not for Eating," was published in *Conscious Choice*. In that year, I also finalized something I called "Critique of Selected Materials Distributed by The Glutamate Association Consumer Education Committee," which I shared with the FDA.

After the *60 Minutes* segment on MSG was aired, no food editor would take my calls. And from that time forward, no major media have even mentioned that MSG might be anything less than safe.

"NO MSG ADDED"

In April 1991, we were exploring the possibility of suing companies that falsely advertised "No MSG," "No Added MSG," or "No MSG Added" on products.

Stouffers, for one, had undertaken a campaign of deceptive and misleading advertising. Stouffers stated on labels that there was no MSG in its Lean Cuisine product line. It used the words "No added MSG" or "No MSG added," but the product contained hydrolyzed protein, which invariably contains MfG. Some of us filed complaints with the Illinois Attorney General. Some filed complaints with the Federal Trade Commission (FTC). Both appeared to be extremely interested. "Deceptive" and "misleading" were words those two offices didn't like. There was hope they could and would do something about the false advertising.

What if the media picked up on it? What if the media told the American public Stouffers had been deceptive and misleading in its advertising? The American public might even come to understand that MSG sensitivity was really sensitivity to all free glutamic acid in all hydrolyzed protein products. To make that happen, we'd have to put considerable effort into writing press releases and sending them to the media. It would be work, yes, but it might be worth the effort.

On July 8, 1991, before we mobilized our efforts, Stouffers called Dr. Schwartz and told him that due to pressure from the FTC, they had withdrawn their "No MSG" claim.

Stouffers wasn't the only company whose deceptive and misleading labeling had come to the attention of public officials. Eleven State Attorneys General, led by Robin Bleecher, Deputy Attorney General from Pennsylvania, felt lawsuits against those who mislabeled products containing MfG would be appropriate. In 1991, in response to lawsuits, consent decrees were entered into by Pepperidge Farm Inc.[45] and Matlaw's Food Products, Inc.[46], and in 1992, a consent decree was entered into by S&B International Corporation[47]. In 1990, Union Foods agreed to pay $153,000 to settle a civil complaint filed by the Ventura County California District Attorney's office[48].

"This is a classic case of false advertising," Ventura County District Attorney Michael Bradbury said in a news release. "It is widely known that many consumers do not want to ingest MSG"[49].

Even the FDA took part in the activity, although not a very big part. It sent Fantastic Foods, Inc. a Regulatory Letter after finding that "The Tomato Vegetable and Curry Vegetable Instant Ramen soups are misbranded as defined in Section 201(n) of the [Food, Drug and Cosmetic Act] since the statement 'NO MSG ADDED' is false and misleading in that the label fails to reveal a material fact, namely that monosodium glutamate (MSG) is added to the product in a significant amount as a natural constituent in the ingredient, hydrolyzed vegetable protein (HVP)"[50].

Federal Food, Drug, and Cosmetic Act. Section 201 (n)

"(n) If an article is alleged to be misbranded because the labeling or advertising is misleading, then in determining whether the labeling or advertising is misleading there shall be taken into account (among other things) not only representations made or suggested by statement, word, design, device, or any combination thereof, but also the extent to which the labeling or advertising fails to reveal facts material in the light of such representations or material with respect to consequences which may result from the use of the article to which the labeling or advertising relates under the conditions of use prescribed in the labeling or advertising thereof or under such conditions of use as are customary or usual."

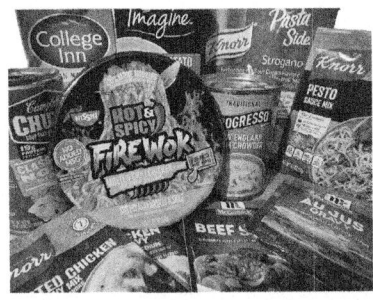

But despite a great deal of activity, nothing much has changed. "No MSG Added" labels continue to proliferate. In 2022, attorneys in California filed a number of class action suits protesting the illegal use of "No MSG," "No MSG added," or "No added MSG" for products that contained MfG.

While all this was going on, we were exploring the possibility of commissioning analyses of MSG-containing products to find out just how much MSG there really was in processed food. We had every reason to believe that figures used by the glutamate industry were unreliable. Looking back, I can't help but wonder why I ever believed anything the Glutes said. They lied in 1990, and are still lying about the amount of MfG in various ingredients, and continue to lie about the amount of

MfG needed to cause an adverse reaction.

1991 — 1992

I found I was writing, often for myself...things I could say to the computer but nowhere else. Private things. Things no one else would ever see. I couldn't tell the world that Jack was mean or angry or irritable, even if it was just when he was exposed to MfG. I couldn't even tell a friend. By this time, we knew our phones were bugged, at least from time to time (our fax machine told us that), so a "secret" never got told on the phone. I could just see someone at Ajinomoto picking up on something I said and using it to discredit Jack. I never bothered to figure out just how they would do that, but I knew they were pros.

Every six months or so, I'd put down my mixing spoons and pencils, turn off the computer and the stove, climb the stairs, flop down on my bed, and have a good cry. No one would ever know that I was frightened, thinking of what the consequences of doing what we were doing might be.

The "Alzheimer's" was gone, or so it seemed, but the signs and symptoms of Alzheimer's, which now could be understood as adverse reactions to MfG, persisted. They appeared every time Jack ingested MfG. Well, not exactly. It's more accurate to say that every time one of those signs or symptoms occurred, careful scrutiny of what Jack had eaten revealed a hidden source of MfG.

We were beginning to understand what Ajinomoto was doing. First, **they** insisted that only double-blind studies could be legitimately used as evidence that people couldn't tolerate MSG. And that's all they had to do. If that was the instruction they gave to the FDA, that became the rule. We didn't yet know that the placebos used in their double-blind studies were chosen to produce the same reactions as those caused by MSG.

Second, they worked to keep consumers in the dark about which processed foods contained MfG and which ones didn't. They'd hide MfG in ingredients that gave no clue to the fact that they contained MfG — ingredients like sodium caseinate, hydrolyzed soy protein, and natural flavoring, for example. That way, consumers would have no way of knowing whether or not there was MfG in products they'd recently eaten.

TRAVELING ABROAD

Outside of the U.S., avoiding MSG wasn't yet a problem. On February 23, 1991, Jack and I flew from Chicago to Kenya and then moved on to Tanzania. From Nairobi, we drove with our group of eight into Tanzania to Lake Manyara and then to the Serengeti National Park — deep in the heart of the savannah on the famous migration corridor. Our group was small, the animals were magnificent, and we had the good fortune of seeing the migration — mile after mile of wildebeests and others strung out across the savannah, including females with little ones in tow.

We had the finest accommodations and the best food available. Sometimes we slept in camping lodges; sometimes we slept in tents. Food was plentiful, good tasting and, for the most part, free of MfG. I don't have to tell you that we'd researched the food situation thoroughly before taking off to this other side of the world. Knorr products were the only thing Jack had to stay away from. That wasn't a problem, since there was plenty of good fresh food prepared without benefit of Knorr bouillon or sauces.

1992

By 1992, we were well versed in the names of ingredients in which MfG was hidden. The food industry hadn't yet embarked on its out-and-out campaign to invent new MfG-containing ingredients with unrecognizable names. At the FDA, nothing had changed, but we were beginning to more easily recognize instances of FDA/industry cooperation.

In January, President George H. W. Bush was taken ill in Japan, not from a typical Japanese meal, but from a U.S.-style meal. We watched his reaction replayed on the television, and it sure looked like an MSG reaction to us. A little MSG with a little wine used to throw Jack into anaphylactic shock before atrial fibrillation replaced anaphylactic shock as his primary reaction. We had to laugh when someone on President Bush's staff told us it couldn't have been MSG-related because Bush was eating American-style food. I'll bet they actually believed that.

Late in the year, I started planning a wedding for our oldest daughter. Jack was adamant about being able to eat at a wedding he was paying for, and that wasn't easy. It seemed that another MfG-containing ingredient was being added to the food supply every other day.

SUGAR

The issue of sugar was interesting. Early on, Jack found that he reacted to some recipes containing sugar, but not all of them. It was clear the amount was very small, because in most cases he'd feel generally bad, but not terrible. By trial and error, backed by great determination, he found he didn't get sick when he used Domino brand sugar, but always got sick when C&H sugar was used.

As it happened, there was a food broker down the hall from Jack's office, and they had become friends. One of his specialties was sugar, and he knew the president of C&H personally.

The C&H president was interested. He couldn't understand why his sugar would be different from others, since raw materials were often procured from the same sources, and the process of making sugar was the same throughout the industry. He did, however, agree to turn the problem over to his laboratory and get back to Jack with an analysis of his sugar. In the end, he wrote that there was a small amount of free glutamic acid in the final sugar product, but no one had a clue as to how it got there. The laboratory chemist said it was so small that no one could possibly react to it.

Actually, "it's such a small amount that no one could possibly react to it" is a basic component of the glutamate industry propaganda program. When consumers call companies that sell products containing MfG but give no clue to its presence, if other diversionary tactics fail, glutamate industry representatives will admit that MfG is in a product, but in such a small amount that no one could possibly react to it. Funny, isn't it, that no one says that about peanuts. No one says that just a little bit of peanut butter or peanut oil couldn't possibly cause a reaction.

CANCER

In August 1992, we attended a meeting of the American Chemical Society in Washington, DC., where the FDA's Dr. Lawrence Lin presented a paper titled "Regulatory Status of Maillard Reaction Flavors." Lin told us that reaction flavors, by virtue of their processing, contain processed free glutamic acid (MfG).[E] He also told us they contain carcinogenic heterocyclic amines[51,52].

Not long after that, we became aware that acid-hydrolyzed proteins contain cancer-causing propanols as well as MfG[53-56]. The FDA has known that since 1990 if not before[57], but aside from suggesting that the levels of carcinogens in acid-hydrolyzed proteins in food be cut down, the FDA has done nothing to limit consumers' exposure, or even to warn them about these carcinogens.

WASHINGTON, DC

Our country's capital is an interesting place for MSG-sensitive people. When forced to eat outside of his own home, and unable to carry something to eat with him, Jack chose to eat in high-end restaurants, believing it would be easier for them to produce meals without using processed food. He found that in Washington, DC, the restaurants that catered to lawmakers used little, if any, MfG.

Problems or not, we continued to travel, but each year became more difficult. Jack's sensitivity to MfG was clearly growing. Increased amounts of MfG were being poured into food without disclosure. The food industry had developed a "clean label" program for hiding MfG, and more processed foods were being used throughout the world, but not as much MfG was being used in Europe or Asia as in the U.S.

THE FDA, BUSINESS AS USUAL

The FDA was operating as it always had on behalf of the glutamate industry. In July 1992, the FASEB report, Safety of Amino Acids Used in Dietary Supplements, was published[58]. We knew that on page 166, we'd find the words:

> "...it is prudent to avoid the use of dietary supplements
> of L-glutamic acid by pregnant women, infants, and
> children...[and] by women of childbearing age and
> individuals with affective disorders"

As we'd come to expect we saw nothing in the press about the toxic potential of MSG.

Sometime in 1992, the FDA appointed both IGTC Chairman Ebert and IGTC spokesperson Kristin McNutt to the spots set aside for consumer representatives in the FDA Food Advisory Committee[59,60]. Were we frustrated? Yes. Discouraged? Sometimes. Relentless? Always.

Having come to the conclusion that the glutamate industry was defrauding the public with full knowledge and approval of the FDA, we asked the FDA/HHS Office of the Inspector General (OIG) to investigate our charge that the behavior of the FDA was inappropriate[61]. In turn, the OIG turned the investigation over to the Office of Research Integrity (ORI)[62] thereby guaranteeing that our petition would be killed. The ORI oversees and directs many Public Health Service research integrity activities on behalf of the Secretary of Health and Human Services, but does not oversee regulatory research integrity activities of the FDA[63]. Therefore, under no circumstances would the ORI have jurisdiction in this matter.

As you might have anticipated, Jack and I next took our concerns to Richard Durban, long-time Senator from Illinois. After all, it is the Congress that funds the FDA. And that, sadly, was where it all died. For the staffer on whom the senator relied for advice on health issues knew, without a doubt, that MSG is perfectly safe. She had the details of Ajinomoto's playbook down word for word.

Admittedly, I've done no study on the subject, but experience in dealing with lawmakers tells me that at least one person in every congressional office has been groomed to understand that MSG is harmless.

As often happened, there was an upside to the contacts I made. When I called the ORI as directed, I had the good luck of speaking to Dr. Richard Broadwell, a neuroscientist who'd taken the job at the ORI for personal reasons. Although he could do nothing for us as an ORI staff member, he was generous in sharing information related to neuroscience, and he taught me a great deal.

D.C. AND THE FDA'S FASEB STUDY

In many ways, 1992 simply ran into 1993, but in fundamental ways, 1993 was different. In 1993, FASEB was shaping a study on the safety of MSG in food, which would eventually become known as the 1995 FASEB Report. The study was commissioned and designed by the FDA, given for execution to FASEB (an organization that had minimal standards for controlling conflicts of interest) and billed as an "independent study"[64]. During most of 1993, commenting on and monitoring the activities of FASEB and its "Expert Panel" occupied us.

As part of the study, a public meeting was scheduled for April 7, 1993. The meeting was advertised as a public forum for submission of scientific data on the safety[F] of MSG.

In February 1993, prior to taking testimony at the public hearing, FASEB published a preliminary report called the Tentative Report[65]. I thought the publication of a preliminary report prior to the public hearing was a pretty clear indication of how meaningless the public's testimony to FASEB would be. I suspect that if a public hearing for this investigation hadn't been required, it would never have occurred.

Thinking back to the Tentative Report and the April open hearing, looking at my notes and then thinking of the contract between the FDA and FASEB, I sometimes wonder why I bothered to participate. The whole thing was a dog-and-pony show from the start, set up to vindicate the use of MSG. The Expert Panel (rife with conflicts of interest) would evaluate "scientific data" that would have been provided by the IGTC, ignore the testimony of those who criticized the studies from which that badly flawed "scientific data" came, and entirely discount the testimony of MSG-sensitive people because they hadn't subjected themselves to double-blind studies to validate their reports of MSG sensitivity. The design of the study, which consisted of 18 questions to be answered by the Expert Panel, was such that under no circumstances would the flavor enhancer called monosodium glutamate be judged to be toxic[66]. Take question 13, for example:

> "Are there any studies conducted [with live subjects] during the 1980s or 1990s that provide additional insight concerning the capacity of orally administered MSG to mediate acute damage (lesions) of the arcuate nucleus of the anterior hypothalamus or of other circumventricular structures in the CNS of nonhuman primates?"

> FASEB's answer? "No. The Expert Panel was unaware of any studies performed within the last 15 years that have directly addressed the ability of orally ingested MSG to produce lesions in nonhuman primates."

The true answer? Studies demonstrating that orally ingested MSG produced lesions in laboratory animals had been so well documented in the 1970s, that researchers had no need to replicate those studies in the 1980s and 1990s, and wouldn't have wasted their time or the lives of laboratory animals doing so[67]. Moreover, had such studies been undertaken, mice, not the more expensive primates, would have been their subjects, for it had previously been demonstrated that mice represent the human condition better than non-human primates[68].

What about the issue of conflicts of interest? The FDA had rules to prohibit them, but they hired FASEB to do the study of the safety of MSG, and FASEB had impotent rules for dealing with conflicts of interest. It has occurred to me more than once that its lax standards for conflicts of interest were likely a major reason the FDA used FASEB so often.

There was no end to the deception that began with the FDA's announcement of the study. There was ample opportunity for us to comment on the chicanery, and we commented each and every time we found an opportunity to do so. On March 26, 1993, for example, I wrote to Kenneth D. Fisher, Ph.D., Director, Life Sciences Research Office FASEB.

"The Tentative Report arrived last week, and I still cannot find the words to adequately express how disappointed I was when I read it. FASEB did not address the question of risk. In fact, FASEB focused on subjects that would obscure the issue."

The response was as it always would be with phrases like, "this is just one piece of the study," or "there will be others added to the panel of experts."

I still quote from Dr. Richard Henneberry's April 7 testimony to FASEB:

"I consider it ironic, that the pharmaceutical industry is investing vast resources in the development of glutamate receptor blockers to protect [central nervous system] neurons against glutamate neurotoxicity in common neurological disorders, while at the same time the food industry, with the blessing of the FDA, continues to add great quantities of glutamate to the food supply"[69].

I felt bad that so many good people traveled to Washington to testify before FASEB, believing their input would have value. Neither they, nor I, realized at the time that there was no chance the final report would even suggest that use of MSG should be meaningfully regulated.

Some people still believe the FDA is charged with safeguarding the health or the nation, but it's my experience that as early as 1990, the FDA was serving as guardian of big business. Not just business. Big Business.

Before we set out for Washington in April, we'd determined that we'd spend a month there, testifying before the three members of the Expert Panel who'd been assigned to listen to testimony in the public hearing, attending the balance of the FASEB meeting, and visiting Congress. We rented an apartment in Chevy Chase, Maryland, close to the metro line, and furniture to go in it.

After Jack found Ebert's statement about the use of aspartame in placebos, we extended our stay in Washington. I wrote to Beatrice Trum Hunter:

"We have been wonderfully busy here in D.C.

"We have spent a good deal of time at the FDA Dockets, reading everything that was submitted to FASEB for the present study.

"We have drawn heavily from those materials in preparing materials to document the hazards caused by MSG. We have started carrying that documentation to meetings with Senators, Representatives, and their staffs. So far everyone has been incredibly receptive."

Again, as always, I was hopeful. In the end, however, the incredibly receptive members of Congress belonged to the wrong party, weren't on the right committee to get anything done with regard to labeling, or were simply overwhelmed at the time with other issues. They'd pass our information on to an MSG-sensitive family member, but would do nothing for their constituents.

ISRAEL

In November, we traveled to Israel with a group from the Chicago chapter of the Weizmann Institute of Science. A number of extremely interesting peer-reviewed studies had been done by Brina Frieder and Veronika Grimm of this respected scientific institute[70,71]. They had demonstrated that prenatal exposure of pregnant rats to MSG in their drinking water resulted in long-lasting changes in general activity level and in the performance of complex discrimination tasks, and resulted in long-term neurochemical modifications in the brains of their offspring.

We knew that MSG ingested by the mother could pass through the placenta to the fetus in utero and affect learning. It was not until 2021, however, that I saw in these data the revelation that pregnant humans who ingested large quantities of MfG in processed and ultra-processed foods would pass those excitotoxic amino acids to their unborn children causing glutamate-induced brain damage in the arcuate nucleus leading to obesity, reproductive dysfunction, behavior disorders and more -- just as Olney had found in animals in 1969 and the years that followed.

It was a thrill and delight to be in the company of the honest and talented scientists of the Weizmann Institute. It was also exciting to travel throughout the marvelous country of Israel, recreating the ancient and experiencing the new.

But in Jack's excitement, he forgot his limitations. We were in an area populated by Hasidic Jews in Jerusalem when he spied a coffee cake in a shop window that was the spitting image of the wonderful cake his mother used to make. For years, he'd looked for his mother's recipe and/or a bakery that produced a similarly wonderful coffee cake, and in Jerusalem he'd found it. He bought two, consuming one cake immediately and the second one as soon as we got back to the hotel.

Bakery goods made for people who keep kosher will very likely be made with margarine rather than butter, and margarine will almost invariably contain MfG. I don't know if it was the margarine, but something in the coffee cake contained MfG, and Jack became exhausted beyond belief and fell into a really foul mood. It was normal for him to suffer extreme fatigue and mood change after ingesting MfG. Overeating doesn't bring on MfG reactions.

TARASOFF AND KELLY

In December 1993, a typical glutamate industry-sponsored study done for the IGTC in Australia by Leonid Tarasoff and Michael Kelly was published in the journal *Food and Chemical Toxicology*[72]. At the time Tarasoff and Kelly were faculty in the Department of Chemistry, Faculty of Business & Technology, University of Western Sydney, Australia. Quite a stretch to have faculty from the Chemistry Department in the Department of Business and Technology doing research on MSG, and interesting to see that the IGTC had gone to Australia for its researchers.

There was nothing special about that study itself. True to form, the subjects claimed to be MSG-sensitive but might not have been so. Researchers counted only a few of the many MSG reactions as such for purposes of the study, only counting them if they occurred within two hours following testing, even though reactions are known to occur as much as 48 hours after ingestion. And, the placebos contained neurotoxic aspartame.

Predictably, I wrote a lengthy letter to the editor of *Food and Chemical Toxicology* detailing the flaws in the Tarasoff and Kelly study -- a letter submitted for publication[73]. On April 6, 1994, Managing Editor Tuan Ho wrote back that my letter to the editor would be published, but on June 1, Editor in Chief J.F. Borzelleca, from the faculty of the Medical College of Virginia where Dr. Donald Kirby was conducting studies for the IGTC[74], wrote to me that "after reconsideration we cannot accept your comments on the paper by Tarasoff and Kelly for publication... Our concern is that your critique could be wrongly exploited by different groups of people involved in the MSG issue..."[75].

What made the Tarasoff and Kelly study so very special was the fact that acceptance of my letter to the editor was followed two months later by its rejection.

When I protested the decision not to publish my letter, Borzelleca personally told me there was no hurry, because the September 1994 FASEB report was being returned to FASEB by the FDA. Borzelleca said he'd seen a copy of the report and knew of discussion between the FDA and glutamate industry about it. That was how I learned that the report of the "independent study" done for the FDA by FASEB had been given to the glutamate industry for review, and, because it hadn't been found satisfactory, was going to be redone.

AMWA

In 1994, I joined the American Medical Writers' Association (AMWA). A good friend on the AMWA governing board had convinced me to join, and I remained a member through 2001. By and large, AMWA members worked for pharmaceutical companies, producing reports of clinical trials, promotional material, or information about the benefits of pharmaceuticals, and I was uncomfortable chit-chatting with people who were proud of the pharmaceutical companies they worked for, and blind to any flaws in their research.

NOMSG

For three days in July, 1994, the NOMSG consumer group held its annual meeting at the Chicago Marriott Downtown. One of our presenters was Dr. Russell Blaylock, who'd recently published the book, *Excitotoxins: The Taste that Kills*, which included a well-researched description of what excitotoxins are, where they're found, and how they react in the body[76]. The excitotoxins in which we were personally interested were the glutamic acid in MSG and the aspartic acid in aspartame.

The meeting was well advertised, given that major newspapers were reluctant to give us coverage. We arranged for participants to earn continuing education credits, which possibly encouraged a few people not sensitive to MfG to attend.

One person who didn't attend was The Glutamate Association's executive director, Richard Cristol. Someone claiming to be from his office had called earlier in the week and asked if he could attend, but he never materialized.

The Marriott provided all the food and drink served at the conference, and I had worked with the restaurant staff to make certain there was nothing served that would cause an MSG-sensitive person to have a reaction. When people began reporting they were having MSG reactions following the conference banquet (one of those people being Jack), it was clear there'd been a problem in the kitchen. When we inquired, we were told that contrary to the standard procedure of keeping at least one meal served at a banquet, all the food we'd been served that night had been destroyed.

Jack and I stayed regularly at Marriott Residence Inns because they provided not only excellent accommodations, but kitchens equipped with cooking utensils. I had been working with the Marriott people in Washington, hoping to convince them to work with us, possibly even sponsor research on MSG toxicity. However following the questionable dinner, NOMSG's president, Kathleen Schwartz became confrontational. And although Jack and I begged her to work with the Marriott people, not against them, to find out how our dinners had become contaminated, Kathleen threatened to call the police and the newspapers and sue the Marriott Corporation. She ended up doing none of that, but any chance we had for future cooperation with Marriott vanished.

THE CHICAGO TRIBUNE

There was more to the NOMSG meeting that spoke of glutamate-industry influence. Jack had contacted the Chicago media and visited some of the local newspapers to encourage them to attend, but only Steve Pratt, food editor of the *Chicago Tribune*, was there.

As he was leaving after the first day, Jack spoke to Pratt and told him he hoped he'd enjoyed the presentations. Pratt responded that he was so impressed with the topic and presenters that he'd already rearranged his schedule and would be returning for the second day. He assured Jack there'd be an article on MSG and our meeting in the food section of the *Tribune* the following Thursday.

On Thursday, there was indeed a sizeable article in the *Tribune's* food section[77]. To our dismay, however, it contained a short paragraph announcing the fact that there'd been a meeting of NOMSG, and Dr. Blaylock had made a presentation in which he described the dangers of MSG. The article then jumped to the fact that Pratt had spoken to Dr. John D. Fernstrom to discuss the subject of MSG, and continued with the sort of misinformation we'd grown to refer to as glutamate industry propaganda.

Jack was furious. Fernstrom had represented the interests of the glutamate industry for many years, and even as of 2022, still did. Jack called Pratt and asked him to explain. While Pratt was polite, he refused to do any correction or retraction. And he wouldn't consider doing another story about MSG.

Not long afterwards, Pratt retired. Some two years later, Jack received a letter in which Pratt apologized for the article he'd written, advising Jack that as an employee of the newspaper, he was sometimes told the direction a given article should take. He commented that he was sure Jack was doing the right thing, and ended by saying Jack should keep up the good work.

Jack had also interacted with the *Chicago Tribune* after release of the *60 Minutes* program about MSG. The "war plan" of the glutamate industry that Jack had received, which was designed to kill the program or do crisis management, had suggested that individuals who had good relationships with reporters should contact them and ask for assurance that articles would appear indicating that MSG is safe and that the MSG segment was nothing more than another Alar-scare staged by *60 Minutes*. Sure enough, following the broadcast the *Chicago Tribune* had published an article indicating that the content of the *60 Minutes* segment was inaccurate and MSG was safe[78]. It had all of the earmarks of a piece written directly by The Glutamate Association, the IGTC, or IFIC.

With the exception of a single article published in 2008[79], the *Chicago Tribune* has never published anything that might indicate MSG is toxic.

The owners of the *Tribune* also owned a major radio outlet, WGN. Jack was contacted by WGN radio personality Kathy O'Malley of the Kathy and Judy show, who suffered from MSG-induced migraine headaches. She invited Jack to be interviewed on the show and take calls.

An initial visit turned into three segments on MSG. At one time, O'Malley interviewed Delores Nick, a woman sensitive to MSG who'd appeared on the *60 Minutes* program. Subsequently, O'Malley told her listeners that in all her years in media, she'd never received as many contacts from listeners as she received while they were doing the segments about MSG. Off the air, she asked that Jack keep her informed about the MSG issue, and contact her when something important came up.

Sometime later, Jack tried to contact O'Malley's producer to tell him about something Jack thought would be of interest to her. Only through Jack's persistence was he finally connected, and then only to hear the producer say that Jack was wasting his time because they'd been directed by management to never again discuss the subject of MSG.

WASHINGTON, DC

In August 1994, we returned to Washington. During that trip, we visited the offices of Senators Barbara Ann Mikulski, Carol Moseley-Braun, Paul Simon, Paul Wellstone, and others. On Thursday, August 18, Jack visited with Dr. Fred Shank at the FDA. On August 24, Jack and I visited Don Grim at Marriott headquarters. The fences that had been broken in July at the NOMSG convention couldn't be mended.

ENZYMES

One of our alternative medicine friends had told us of a developer, Burton Goldberg, who had amassed a considerable sum of money and decided to use his wealth teaching others all he knew about alternative medicine. Earlier in the year, Goldberg, who had published what he called the ultimate book on alternative medicine[80], joined us at our home for dinner. He believed Jack's MSG problem could be resolved, and suggested that Jack visit Lita Lee, an expert on the use of enzymes.

Jack had been introduced to alternative medicine years ago when a homeopathic physician diagnosed and remedied a condition suffered by one of our children. Allopathic physicians had failed to treat her condition effectively, and Jack was open to Goldberg's suggestion. Moreover, Lee believed taking the enzymes she recommended would help him.

Recognizing his extreme sensitivity, Lee gave him only enough enzymes to use for a couple of weeks to see what their effect might be. However, after three or four days, Jack began to manifest symptoms of MfG toxicity: inability to find the right words when he spoke, loss of balance, disorientation, and a general feeling of being ill. As his symptoms seemed to get worse each day he called Lee, and they agreed he should stop taking the enzymes. She apologized that she wasn't able to help him.

Shortly thereafter, Jack ran into a detail man for a specialty supplement company who understood his reaction to the enzymes. He knew that supplements his company sold were derived from vegetables, and those who manufactured enzymes wouldn't go to the expense of removing all protein before processing. The remaining protein would, therefore, be broken down during production, resulting in the production of free glutamic acid, i.e., MfG.

THE TRUTH IN LABELING CAMPAIGN

In October 1994, Jack, George Bucic, and I incorporated the Truth in Labeling Campaign (TLC) as an Illinois not-for-profit corporation. Kathleen Schwartz of NOMSG had been reluctant to have her consumer group participate in the lawsuit Jack and I were considering, and we decided that to help us move forward in whatever direction we chose to move, we should establish this new organization without membership, so as not to compete with NOMSG.

Toward the end of the year, Jack took a call from a man who introduced himself as Patrick Dilling, a lawyer who claimed to be sensitive to MSG. Dilling wanted to "sue the sons of bitches" over their failure to protect consumers. He called us to secure assistance -- and generate cash to pay his legal fees and out-of-pocket expenses.

THE LAWSUIT

Dilling sued the FDA in the U.S. District Court in St. Louis, in part because St. Louis would be a convenient location for Olney, who'd gladly consented to be a plaintiff. Unfortunately, we didn't take into account the fact that Monsanto, the company that owned aspartame at the time, had its headquarters in St. Louis.

On December 13, 1994, prior to filing the lawsuit, and as required by law, a Citizen Petition that I wrote was filed with the U.S. Department of Health and Human Services, FDA, asking the FDA to require labeling of all MSG found in processed foods. In 1994, there was no distinction being made between the ingredient called monosodium glutamate (MSG) and its excitotoxic component manufactured free glutamic acid (MfG).

I can think of nothing more important to the glutamate industry than preventing identification of MfG wherever and whenever it is used in processed food. After all, if identified, consumers might be able to determine if products containing MfG were causing adverse reactions. It seems to me that in actuality, the fight against identifying MfG in processed foods is tantamount to admission of MfG's toxicity. Think about it. If MSG and MfG weren't harmful, why would they be hidden?

Preparation for suing the FDA was no small matter. There were lawyers to educate, plaintiffs to convince to participate, and press releases to send out. There was also co-counsel to be identified in St. Louis, because Dilling was not licensed to practice law in Missouri. That job fell to us, too.

IMPURITIES

At the end of 1994 we were still learning. We knew Jack would get sick following ingestion of MSG, but not from the glutamate in unadulterated protein, but we still didn't know why. We found our lack of knowledge in this area particularly distressing because the Glutes were getting mileage out of claiming that no one could possibly react to MSG without also reacting to tomatoes and mushrooms, because tomatoes and mushrooms were loaded with glutamate.

It was in 1995 that we learned that the free glutamic acid in an unadulterated tomato is chemically different than the free glutamic acid that occurs in food as a consequence of a manufacturing process[81].

The initial revelation had come from reading a study done in 1994 by Kimber Rundlett and Daniel Armstrong of the Department of Chemistry at the University of Missouri, Rolla: "Evaluation of free D-glutamate in processed foods." According to the study abstract:

> "Monosodium glutamate (MSG) is added to many processed foods at significant levels for flavor enhancement. It is also naturally occurring at high levels in some foods. The enantiomeric composition of free glutamate in foods was examined and all processed foods analyzed were found to contain D-glutamate"[12].

It had taken us more than five years to see what had just become obvious. There is no processed (manufactured) free glutamic acid without impurities.

There are basically three different grades of raw materials used in products:

- Pharmaceutical Grade meets pharmaceutical standards,

- Food Grade meets standards set for human consumption, and

- Feed Grade meets standards set for animal consumption.

The difference between each grade type is one of quality and purity. In technical terms, no substance is 100 percent pure[82]. There will always be unwanted byproducts of production, and there may be substances added to products. The difference between the grades is one of how much of these other substances, these impurities, are present in the product. No free glutamic acid can be produced without simultaneously producing impurities.

The Food Chemical Codex (FCC), which employs these definitions, is a compendium of internationally recognized standards for the purity and identity of food ingredients, including food-grade chemicals, processing aids, foods (such as vegetable oils, fructose, whey, and amino acids), flavoring agents, vitamins, and functional food ingredients (such as lycopene, olestra, and short chain fructooligosaccharides)[83].

On the subject of monosodium glutamate, Yoshi-hisa Sugita, CEO of the IGTC in 1994 (possibly Ebert's replacement), wrote,

> "Specifications of MSG 'not less than 99.0%' means that the 99.0% is the minimum content guaranteed to the user. The actual purity of MSG is around 99.8%, with a small amount of moisture (water lost on drying), and negligible amounts of calcium, organic acids and amino acids"[84].

The food, dietary supplements, and pharmaceuticals that contain manufactured glutamate (glutamate with impurities) cause brain lesions, endocrine disorders and adverse reactions in an undetermined portion of the population. When Olney and others found brain lesions and endocrine disorders in laboratory animals[85], they were using monosodium glutamate purchased in grocery stores in place of what would have been more expensive pharmaceutical-grade glutamic acid[86] (which would also have contained impurities).

RESEARCHERS FOR HIRE

I called Dr. Armstrong and found he was receptive to the idea of doing research for us. He asked only that we cover the expenses of the laboratory assistant(s) who'd be working on the study. We hesitated to give him the go-ahead for what would be a $15,000 personal obligation, and when I called a few days later to accept his research offer, Dr. Armstrong would no longer take my calls.

This was the second time an agreement to do research, agreed to over the phone, had run amuck. The first incident happened in 1993, when researchers in the sleep clinic at Baylor College of Medicine agreed to study the possible effects of MSG on disruptive sleep. Max Hirshkowitz, Ph.D. and Nilgun Gokcebay, M.D. were working with me to design the sleep study when, without notice, they stopped calling me, and stopped taking my calls. So it was with particular interest that we later noted that in 1998, the International Symposium on Glutamate, held in Bergamo, Italy, was sponsored jointly by the Baylor College of Medicine, the Center for Nutrition at the University of Pittsburgh School of Medicine, the Monell Chemical Senses Center, the International Union of Food Science and Technology, and the Center for Human Nutrition. Financial support was provided by the IGTC[87].

BUILDING ON THE BIG LIE

In 1995, consumers had more to contend with than deceptive and misleading labeling and the fact that the FDA was beholden to industry. In response to consumers' inquiries, food companies were lying about the presence of MSG in their products. In one of my articles, I wrote:

> "MSG sensitive people tell numerous stories of being given false and misleading information about MSG by food companies, and of being treated poorly when they attempt to discuss the MSG issue. Certain food companies apparently believe that it is part of their job to keep consumers from knowing what they are eating. Ajinomoto, the world's leading producer of MSG, has run advertisements in food industry magazines suggesting

to food producers that 'disodium inosinate,' a product that works synergistically with MSG, 'can be added in products already containing artificial flavor without changing the label.'"

Most MSG-sensitive individuals who've inquired of food companies about MSG content in products have been told more than once that if they were MSG sensitive, they wouldn't be able to tolerate tomatoes because unadulterated tomatoes contain free glutamic acid just like MSG does. The food companies never mention the impurities that accompany manufactured/processed free glutamic acid (MfG).

LAWSUIT

On August 29, 1995, TLC and 29 independent citizens filed suit in federal court in St. Louis (Truth in Labeling vs. Shalala) represented by Kirkpatrick W. Dilling and Goldstein and Price L.C. asking the court to intercede on their behalf and require that all MSG/MfG in processed foods be labeled[88]. On March 30, 1998, Magistrate Thomas C. Mummert, III dismissed the case.

As plaintiffs, we had to prove the FDA had been "arbitrary and capricious" in its refusal to require that all MSG in processed food be identified on the labels of the products that contained it. Proof of the FDA being arbitrary and capricious lay in the files of the FDA. We knew what it was and we knew where it was, but the FDA refused to release that material to the court when it was requested under discovery. We explained to Magistrate Mummert that in presenting the court with several boxes of irrelevant files in place of the documents requested, the FDA had selectively omitted relevant files and correspondence from the period being reviewed. When challenged, the FDA replied that it had gone through its files and had only sent those that were relevant. The FDA didn't provide the court with a copy of the 1994 FASEB report that had been returned by the FDA to FASEB at the suggestion of Ajinomoto or the IGTC, or copies of information/studies sent to the FDA by Dr. Olney. Magistrate Mummert raised no objection, and our case was closed.

The court's decision said nothing about the safety or toxicity of monosodium glutamate or other MfG-containing ingredients.

Did someone get to Magistrate Mummert? Might the fact that Monsanto had a presence in St. Louis, or the fact that Ajinomoto might have supplied the aspartic acid and phenylalanine ingredients for Monsanto's aspartame have had anything to do with it? Ajinomoto did manufacture both those amino acids and was involved in two joint ventures with Monsanto in the sweetener business in Europe. Interesting questions, but we're still waiting for a whistleblower to come forward with answers.

In 1985, Monsanto had purchased G.D. Searle, the company that invented and first manufactured aspartame, and the aspartame business became a separate Monsanto subsidiary called the NutraSweet Company[89]. Ajinomoto acquired its aspartame business from Monsanto in 2000[90].

LEARNING, ALWAYS LEARNING

It was 1995 and the Glutes were still at it. They seem to have developed a playbook for deceptive practices. In 1995, it was an attempt to discredit one of us.

On August 30, Jack called Dr. Roland Auer, pro-MSG advocate and former member of the FASEB Expert Panel, spending more than an hour on the phone with him, discussing the safety of monosodium glutamate, an issue on which they disagreed. Auer had been appointed to the FASEB Expert Panel as a neuroscientist, possibly to placate Olney, who'd repeatedly commented that in all the FDA's deliberations, no neuroscientist had participated in the FDA's "independent" reviews of MSG safety[91]. As an Expert Panel member, Auer was among those who had found for FASEB that MSG was safe. After the July 1995 FASEB report was published, he and Jack had been interviewed together by Eugenia Halsey for CNN, Auer representing the point of view of the glutamate industry, while Jack represented people who believed MSG was toxic. Not considering that he might be under the spell of the glutamate people, Jack called to provide Auer with information Jack believed he'd overlooked.

Jack thought their conversation had been a simple discussion of an issue on which two people disagreed. He'd shared his ideas freely, without thought that what he said might be misquoted. He'd not yet learned all there was to learn about the way the Glutes operate.

A few days after their conversation, Jack received a seven-page letter from Auer. It was a gross misrepresentation of what Jack had said over the phone. In essence, Auer had taken Jack's comments out of context and then sent copies of his letter to people who might be interested in discrediting Jack. I'd seen this tactic used by the glutes previously, and I would see it again: write something destructive about your target, which later the Glutes will quote from as though the distortions of the writer were fact.

Periodically, I would receive a phone call or letter from someone who was clearly an agent of the IGTC (or Ajinomoto). Sometimes the contacts came from students "writing a paper" and looking for information, who often were not registered at the colleges they claimed to be attending. Some came with criticism of our lawsuit or our website, spewing out invectives for no apparent reason — wasting our time, possibly attempting to upset us.

To me, Auer was just a different version of the same thing. His spin seemed to be to repeat some of what Jack said, out of context, cast in a form that could later be used by the Glutes to discredit him. The Glutes seem to have a special talent for doing such things. They really are good at what they do.

Drs. Ronald Simon and Donald Stevenson, then affiliated with Scripps Clinic and Research Foundation, La Jolla, California, were also part of the 1995 phenomenon. On the day before the August 31, 1995 FASEB report to the FDA was released to the public, they wrote to inform the FDA that they believed the FASEB report had made a grave error in stating that MSG was known to be an asthma trigger[92]. They didn't mention the fact that in 1995, they were doing research for the IGTC.

1995 — 1996

In 1995, Jack and I were dividing time between San Diego and Chicago, with trips to Washington on occasion. To the best of our knowledge, our phones were still bugged, our fax machines suffered intercepted transmissions, at least from time to time, and we knew better than to say anything that might prove useful to the Glutes either at home or in the car. We laughed about our secrets being secret. There wasn't a whole lot more to laugh about.

We ate out only on rare occasion, as Jack had become acutely sensitive to the smallest amounts of MfG, and none of the MfG in processed food was labeled as such. Friends didn't invite us for dinner, because they knew Jack wouldn't eat, and they didn't like to come to our house for dinner because they knew they couldn't reciprocate. When we went to our children's homes, we brought our own food or did all the shopping and cooking. When we traveled in the U.S., we had an electric hot plate and portable electric cooler with us, and timed our travel to stay at a Residence Inn that offered rooms with kitchens. If a restaurant meal couldn't be avoided, Jack ordered a steak with no seasoning made in a pan cleaned before the cooking began.

When we traveled in Europe — and I'm talking of 20-25 years ago — Jack rarely had a problem. He ate fresh fruits and vegetables and unadulterated fish, meat, and poultry; soup made from scratch without benefit of bouillon cubes and flavor enhancers, and ate cheese and ice cream made from whole milk that hadn't been ultra-pasteurized.

Toward the end of the year, the pace of MSG-related activities slowed considerably. FASEB had turned in a report to the IGTC's liking[93]. Magistrate Mummer would refuse to order that the FDA provide all relevant material we'd asked for under discovery, so even before the verdict was in, we knew we'd lost the case against the FDA. Celebrities like Dean Edell and Julia Child were being recruited by the IGTC or The Glutamate Association to speak positively about the glories of monosodium glutamate. And the clean label industry was booming.

STANFORD UNIVERSITY HOSPITAL

At 8:30 a.m. on October 17, 1996, Jack reported to Stanford University Hospital for prostate cancer treatment. He was involved in what he thought to be routine intake procedures when a "crash cart" appeared with staff in tow, and Jack was taken to cardiac care and hooked up to a cardiac monitor.

"What are you doing?" He asked the nurse. "I'm here for prostate cancer treatment."

"No confusion," said the nurse, "but we have to evaluate the seriousness of your atrial fibrillation before we proceed."

Jack had no idea he was fibrillating, but once known, it wasn't hard to figure out where it had come from. He'd recently brought his high blood pressure under control using a pharmaceutical called procardia, and one of its possible side effects was atrial fibrillation[94]. Once compromised by a susceptibility to atrial fibrillation, he'd now fibrillate each time he ingested MfG.

In the past, Jack had suffered from fatigue and mood changes when ingesting MfG, and had gone into anaphylactic shock when ingesting MfG with alcohol. His cardiologist didn't think fibrillating was a step up from going into anaphylactic shock. He suggested Jack would likely die from the stress placed on his heart by repeated atrial fibrillation — if a particular attack in and of itself didn't kill him. Since increased risk for cardiac arrest and stroke are side effects of fibrillation, Jack didn't think fibrillation was a step in the right direction, either. It ordinarily took alcohol in combination with MfG to bring on anaphylactic shock. Atrial fibrillation came on after ingesting MfG without the help of alcohol.

We spent three months at Stanford. Jack would go to the hospital in the morning, return home and, at my insistence, take a nap — whether he was tired or not. Afternoons and weekends were spent doing the things that tourists might routinely do: shopping, touring, and going to the opera in San Francisco. Our afternoons also included shopping for and making dinner.

NAET

On May 19, 1997, a young alternative medicine doctor practicing in Chicago came to one of the NOMSG meetings to tell us about a procedure he thought might be of value to MSG-sensitive people. The procedure had been created by Dr. Devi Nambudripad, who'd come from India as a nurse and gone on to become an acupuncturist and chiropractor. She called her procedure Nambudripad's Allergy Elimination Technique (NAET)[95,96]. Among other things, it involved the use of muscle strength testing, known as applied kinesiology.

The demonstration was poorly presented and difficult to follow. No one at our small meeting saw anything of value. It was only years later that we learned we were wrong.

THE INSTITUTE OF FOOD TECHNOLOGISTS

In June 1997, Jack and I attended the Institute of Food Technologists (IFT) annual meeting in Orlando. I had joined the IFT in 1993 after

attending one of its meetings in Chicago. The idea for joining had
come from Ellen Metzger, who'd been in Chicago at the time. Ellen was
MSG-sensitive and interested in raising the public's awareness of the
adverse effects MSG could have on health and well-being. Ellen had all
kinds of good ideas.

In addition to dropping in on presentations that interested us, we
joined a luncheon session at which the FDA's Dr. Shank was speaking,
and a dinner hosted by *Food Chemical News*. Most of our time, however,
was spent on the exhibition floor, for we knew we still had much to learn.
It was there that I approached a youngish looking fellow standing in the
booth of an analytical testing laboratory and asked him if his company
would analyze MSG for me.

"Absolutely" he responded. "What kind of results would you like us to
give you?" With further discussion, it became clear that through setting
up limits in their testing procedures and defining "MSG" as we desired,
they'd be able to say anything about our MSG sample we wanted them
to say. They'd do that for us — which suggested that industry figures for
amounts of MSG in ingredients and/or products might be meaningless.

COLORADO

The next time we passed through Colorado, we made it our business
to visit the Colorado Historical Society and journey up to Greeley. In
1993, Russell Phares, a former MSG production worker, had written
to FASEB to inquire if they might have some information concerning
"MSG poisoning" that, he said, had been the fate of workers in the Great
Western Sugar factory producing monosodium glutamate. We found his
letter in the FDA docket pertaining to the FASEB study, and wrote to
him.

Eventually, we met Phares, who told us he'd once worked at a
monosodium glutamate production plant in Greeley, cleaning the vats in
which monosodium glutamate was made. He said that eventually both
he and a friend who'd worked with him began having medical problems.
For Phares, it was years of an uncontrollable skin condition and other
problems he wasn't comfortable talking about. He'd become homeless,
but had eventually been taken in by a religious organization where some
of his difficulties had been resolved. Being extremely skillful, Phares lived

at the religious center working as a handyman. He said his friend was living on the streets.

We started at the public library in Greeley, but found little of interest outside of the librarian. She knew nothing of a monosodium glutamate plant, but was happy to share all she knew about Great Western Sugar, and she searched her files for us. The old-timers were all gone, she told us, and she couldn't think of anyone to suggest we talk to.

From what we could gather from the few records we could find, the monosodium glutamate plant had been closed ahead of the closing of the Great Western Sugar plant itself, which would have taken place some years later. One report said the monosodium glutamate plant had been converted to production of a different chemical. Another said it had been bulldozed, records and all, and the rubble carried away. The second option is much more dramatic, the stuff that mystery novels are made of. What actually happened? We don't know.

PARIS

In December 1997, we visited Paris for the second time, not having been there since 1984, before Jack had realized he was sensitive to MfG. His MfG reactions had been increasing in number and severity, leaving him to recover over a period of time while he continued to fibrillate and just didn't feel well. So I made sure we'd be in a location where I could go walking if I had to go walking alone, and we'd be in a place where English was spoken in case Jack needed medical attention.

There was this incredibly cheap airfare, and Jack was so very sure he could eat in Paris, as he used to without getting sick, that I made a few phone calls, found a hotel, and booked our flight.

As Jack said, it's very hard being alive when you have to give up living. I found it hard, too. Waiting for him to eat some bit of processed food that he once ate without reaction. Living in fear that he would be struck down again at any moment. Then living in fear that he wouldn't recover. Sometimes, I would wish it was over, while praying that it never happens.

We had scheduled dinners for every other evening: Apicius on Tuesday, Le Bourdonnais on Thursday, Le Duc on Saturday, and Arpege on Monday — restaurants run by talented chefs who used whole fresh food and had no need for MfG. We wandered the streets, going to new places and seeing new things without ignoring our favorite outdoor food markets, the Rodin Museum, and the Musée d'Orsay.

With Christmas in the air, we sought out the Marché de Noel de Paris, where we found a stall selling an attractive assortment of homemade jams and jellies, some of which contained no pectin.

Pectin is one of the many ingredients that contain MfG. Most jellies and some jams in the United States contain pectin. But there was no pectin in the jam at the Marché de Noel de Paris. Problem was that when we left the market, Jack picked up a jar of jelly, thinking it was jam; the alcohol in the wine that he had been drinking exacerbated the atrial fibrillation caused by the MfG in the pectin in the jelly, and when he made himself a sandwich, he collapsed.

While Jack lay in bed, hopefully recovering, I was writing. I was talking to the computer. There was no one else to talk to, and I had to do something to stem the tide of tears.

It's five in the morning Paris time — and I'm hiding. Hiding behind words. Words that pretend there's a difference between wars played with guns and landmines aimed at changing a country's internal political structure or physical boundaries and wars for power played with unsafe food and drugs, herbicides and pesticides, nuclear power plants and atomic generators, toxic waste dumps, decimated forests and rain forests, all sold to the public as the insignificant fallout of "progress." All sold to improve some corporation's bottom line and to enhance the power of the men and women who openly run the corporations and, I'd guess, probably run the world.

So I write down words, words no one will read, because the men and women who openly run the corporations also run the vehicles through which my words would be transmitted to others — if they were transmitted to others. They're directors of newspaper chains or media conglomerates. If not that, they sit waiting to withhold their advertising dollars from those newspaper chains or media conglomerates that would dare think to defy them and print the words of "food terrorists."

Yes, we've been called that. Maybe that's because we strike terror in the hearts of the men and women who run the corporations that produce the potentially toxic food additives that cause infants to suffer neuroendocrine disorders such as obesity and reproductive disorders (not immediately discernable), cause immediate reactions such as asthma, migraine headache, cardiac tachycardia, depression, nausea and vomiting, seizures, and cardiac arrhythmia; speed, if not cause, the progress of neurodegenerative conditions such as Alzheimer's disease and Amyotrophic lateral sclerosis (ALS) and cause cancer. Yes, cancer-causing heterocyclic amines, monochloro propanols, and dichloro propanols are produced under certain conditions when some forms of MSG are made.

It may be all over in the morning. Jack may be dead, but chances are he'll be alive and well and ready to take on another day in Paris. And if he is — alive and well — I wonder what he'll eat today. A banana, for sure. Probably bread and butter, but not the bread we got at the food market yesterday, since it might have been more than just the jelly that did him in. It might have been the bread or one of the cheeses from the market or even a few leaves of lettuce he munched on from the supply I'd bought for myself. It might even have been that the pastries he had earlier in the day added to his problem.

We'll never know, because Jack isn't going to clone himself and do a series of double-blind studies designed to determine that MfG is safe like Ebert says he must if others are to believe he reacted to the pectin. Ebert would say Jack is really just an anecdote. "Not the food, at all." Or, "Jack probably overdid it carrying heavy packages."

Ebert says there's really no evidence that MSG makes people sick. And he should know, because he gets paid directly by the IGTC, an organization with a secret membership led by the world's greatest producer of the chemicals that go into MSG, a company called Ajinomoto. Directly or indirectly, Ebert has friends in high places like the FDA, the U.S. Department of Agriculture, the American Dietetic Association, the Berkeley Wellness Newsletter, the Association of

Family Physicians, the World Health Organization, the European Communities, and the National Institute of Nutrition out of Ottawa, Canada — just to name a few. Ebert is also a well-respected member of the Institute of Food Technologists (IFT), the people who design chemical concoctions that are passed off as food. Everyone knows that he's a toxicologist. He and his friend Steve Taylor, who also belongs to the IFT and works for the IGTC from his office at the University of Nebraska, assure all their friends at the IFT that MSG is safe. Doesn't it make sense that those who make money from using the product would believe them?

It's six in the morning Paris time. I wonder when Jack will be up and ready to take on the day. I wonder if the sun will shine today, or ever.

CHAPTER FOUR NOTES

A. "Glutes," members of the glutamate industry.

B. Hydrolysis is a chemical process used for breaking down various substances including proteins. When proteins are broken into their component parts, glutamic acid (processed free glutamic acid) is released.

C. A placebo is an inactive substance or preparation used as a control in an experiment or test to determine the effectiveness of a medicinal drug.

D. All the double-blind studies that claim to support the notion that monosodium glutamate is safe for human consumption acknowledge that the IGTC played a role in producing them.

E. Reaction flavors, also known as process flavors, have traditionally been produced by heating a protein source with a sugar source to produce a mixture of chemicals containing flavor value.

F. The word "toxicity" is never mentioned where it might be associated with MSG.

Chapter Five

Jack (In His Own Words)

N ot everyone is sensitive to MSG, at least not as sensitive as I am. Maybe I was brain damaged the time the car was totaled, or the time I was blown up in the boat.

I don't remember much about my early years. When I was born, my parents lived in a small house on the south side of Chicago near present-day Midway Airport. My father, who was born and raised in St. Louis, had dropped out of school after fourth grade to help support his family. As a teenager, he'd built a thriving poultry business, but wanting to better himself, he'd moved to Chicago, where a relative would train him to be a butcher. It was in Chicago that he met my mother. They were married on January 4, 1929. My sister was born on August 18, 1930, and I followed on April 26, 1935.

Not long after I was born, we moved to a two-flat apartment. I remember the apartment and Mrs. Zimmer, who owned the building and lived upstairs. She was a wonderful lady who treated me to yummy cookies and big cold glasses of delicious milk. She said it was just like the milk I refused to drink at home, delivered by the same milkman. But I could tell the difference.

I also remember my grandmother, a wonderful grandmother married to cranky old Grandpa Felix. My father and grandfather had discussions more than once on the subject of children playing at our house. These were discussions, not arguments. There were never arguments in our house. But try as he might, my father couldn't convince Grandpa Felix that if everyone played at our house, even if they made a mess, my mother would know where I was and who I was playing with, and that knowledge was priceless.

It was a rare blood disease that eventually did in Grandpa Felix. Long after he died, my mother preached that I was going to have the same disease because I, like my grandfather, wouldn't eat vegetables.

I didn't drink much milk, either. I really didn't like it. The exceptions were chocolate milk, and the delicious white Wanzer milk served by Mrs. Zimmer. What I really liked was meat. Red meat. I was always a big protein eater. I also liked the bukta (a bohemian coffee cake), cinnamon rolls, streusel-covered coffee cake, and apple strudel my mother baked on Saturday for breakfast on Sunday. I've never found a bukta as wonderful as hers, but I never gave up looking, and tasting.

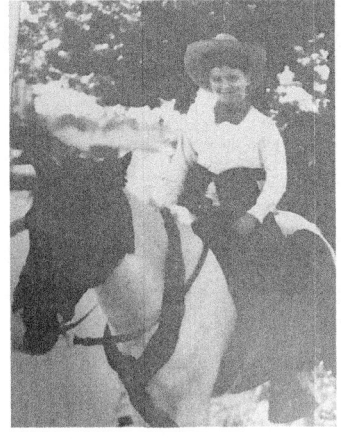

I must have been four years old when my parents bought an empty lot on Winchester Avenue in north Beverly Hills on the south side of Chicago. There were no streetlights. There was no public transportation. The closest house was two blocks away. My father had always wanted to live on a farm where my sister could have a horse and I could have a pony. My mother was definitely a city person. I guess this was a compromise.

The lots behind our house were still empty when I started school. I walked both ways as everyone did, for the idea of special buses to take children to school hadn't yet occurred to anyone. The total enrollment of my school was just about 300 pupils; classes were small and school was fun.

I had a lot of friends and I played a lot of sports. A half block from our house was an overgrown field owned by the school district that we made into a baseball field. Jimmy Finkleton's parents allowed that we could use their push lawn mower to clear the field if we wanted to; and since none of the other kids could push the mower, I cut out the baseball field.

I was in many fights, none of which I started, and none of which I lost. My father had made it very clear that he never wanted to hear that I hit someone, or that I started a fight, but if someone pushed me, I could certainly push that person back. As long as I didn't start the fight, he wasn't opposed to my winning. He and my mother also made me aware that some people are prejudiced. My father told me that if people picked on me for no other reason than being prejudiced, that gave me the right to hit them.

I was just starting 8th grade when my father's doctor suggested that my father retire and take a lengthy trip to relax and rid himself of the pressures of business. My sister had started college, so my parents decided that for a full semester they would go to Florida and I would go with them.

I remember seeing signs in front of hotels that said no Jews or blacks allowed, and as we got deeper into the south, they were more prevalent. My father used to talk about how terrible this was. He pointed out that if we were driving late into the evening and had to find a hotel, we could lie about being Jewish and get a bed. But a black person couldn't walk into that hotel and convince staff that he wasn't black.

In the South, we'd go into grocery stores and see drinking fountains painted a particular pink/brown color for black people to use. To this day, the color brown bothers me. A major portion of the report I did for school that year focused on the prejudice we found in the South.

My father was a remarkable person. Hard work, compassion, and integrity defined the man. I built my life on the lessons he taught me through word and example. He taught me all I know about judging people. He taught me that certain features told volumes about a person. When I had my first assignment in hospital administration, the personnel director would interview potential key employees and have the best three candidates interviewed by the administrators, which included me. He claimed that while he asked most people to talk to candidates to rate them, I listened to the sounds of their voices, looked for certain features, and read the bumps on their heads. History showed that I made the best selections. My father taught me that.

As a child, if I'd come home injured, my father would ask, "Where does it hurt?" If I pointed to my leg, he'd say, "Well, that's very far from your heart. I think you'll be all right."

We were taught never to lie. I can hear his words as though he was speaking today. "Don't ever lie, cause if you lie, sometime later on someone will ask you the same question and you'll have to remember what the lie was. If you tell the truth, it's very easy to remember."

Finally, he would say, "Everyone puts his pants on one leg at a time. As long as you have something to say and are not lying, go up to people and say what you have to say. They might not like you at the time, but they'll respect you for it."

I was 14 years old when I entered Calumet High School. Now, I couldn't walk home for lunch, and there was this thing called homework, which I'd never done before. I liked school all right. There wasn't anything I didn't like at the time except vegetables. Anyhow, if things weren't just as I thought they should be, I could make improvements.

I did well in school with little or no effort. When teachers gave out homework before the end of class, I would finish my assignments before class was over.

The year before graduation, after taking the course exams, I was number two in the class. As soon as I realized I had good enough grades to go to college, I slacked off. I was number 16 when I graduated.

In my second or third year of high school, my mother developed a uterine tumor and became gravely ill. She was so bad that my father had me live with the Berman's, distant relatives, at their summer cottage on Pistake Lake until my mother recovered. At Pistake Lake, I'd go fishing every day with Mr. Berman.

My father liked Pistake Lake, and saw that I liked it, too. "Soon you're going to be out of high school and will be drafted into the army, and who knows, might get killed. So you might as well enjoy yourself, and I'm going to go out there and buy a property."

After the house was built, I'd take my mother to Pistake Lake to measure for curtains, furniture, and such. The last time we made the trip, the road to the house from the main road was covered with ice, and a car speeding toward us hit us head on. In truth, I don't remember what happened after that. I do know I lost consciousness, and I remember seeing a gaping hole in the other car's hood and motor compartment. I also remember that our car was barely moveable—that we made it home very slowly, turning left when necessary, but not able to turn right.

Years later, it came to me that it might have been that accident that set me up for MSG sensitivity. A blow to the head? Damage to the blood brain barrier that is supposed to keep MfG from flowing freely into the brain?

Summers I worked at the local A&P as a meat cutter, working there through my four years of college. I'd cut meat, go home for dinner and go out fishing. On one exceptionally hot day, just before starting college, I gassed up our mahogany Chris Craft before dinner, realizing only too late that the pump registered more gas than the boat's gas tank would hold. I assumed the overflow had gone into the lake, when in truth the bulk of it had gone under the floorboards. Not knowing that, I returned home, docked at the pier, quickly went in to eat dinner, and returned to the boat with my sister and father to go fishing.

I remember pressing the start button. The next thing I remember was waking up and not being able to see anything because there were things on me, and the entire perimeter of the boat was on fire.

I shoved my father off from on top of me, shook off the debris that had been under him, and saw Mr. Berman from six houses down, running. Mr. Berman never ran. My mother was on the front porch screaming, "They're dead, they're dead," and the dog was barking. Moving my father woke him up, and the two of us got out of the boat together. To this day, I don't know how we did it. I had a perfect shave on one side of my face, and my eyelashes and eyebrows were gone on that side, too. I had a rather deep cut on the little finger of my left hand. The steering wheel I'd been holding was folded in half, the glass windshield was entirely missing, and my mother was screaming that my sister was still in the boat. She lay unconscious in the back with lipstick smeared across her face, giving the impression that her whole face was on fire.

"Quick. Get a bucket of water, there's fire," my father commanded as he pulled my sister from the boat. So I ran to the pump at the back of the house, and pumped a bucket of water to bring to the lake and the burning boat. The lake? I'd brought a bucket of water to the lake.

It was shortly after the boat explosion that I took my placement exams at Northwestern. I might just as well have stayed at home, because mentally I was absent.

I knew nothing about applying to college. My best friend, Herb, was applying to Northwestern, and we'd agreed that we would live together. Somehow, I got an application and filled it out. I didn't apply to any other school. It never occurred to me that I might not be accepted.

For my first two years at Northwestern, I lived in Sargent Hall, a relatively new high-rise dormitory. Herb had joined a fraternity that didn't accept Jews. Eventually, I moved with Dick, my roommate, to a newly renovated dormitory (that was actually not quite finished), and immediately found that we were uncomfortably cold at night. After protesting to the university a number of times without getting their attention, I found the home phone number of the dean and called him. Every night in the middle of the night I called the dean, gave him my name, told him where we lived, and explained that while he was comfortable in his nice warm bed, we were freezing. Remarkably, after the third day, or should I say third night of phone calls, a heating crew showed up and the issue was resolved.

College was generally unremarkable. I was a biology major and became so interested in genetics that I took independent study with a genetics professor.

My father had wanted me to be a physician, but I couldn't stand blood. Instead, I looked into hospital administration. I visited hospitals to see what the administrators were doing. I visited with two administrators whom I found to be inadequate, and determined that I could easily do better than they did. I had to take some business courses, but they were easy.

Except for the prom in high school, I didn't date, and I wasn't much more aggressive in college until Dick fixed me up with Tena Ross, a University of Illinois coed.

Down the road, I applied to Northwestern's program for hospital administration. My two greatest challenges were convincing the faculty that my age wouldn't be a detriment to becoming a successful hospital administrator, and that I could find employment in a world where Jewish administrators were a rarity.

I graduated in June 1957. Shortly thereafter, Tena and I were married. I had a part-time job in the credit department at Weiss Memorial Hospital and Tena worked for an obstetrician, preparing and reading pap smears.

After a year of intensive coursework, field trips, and lectures, I accepted a residency at Mount Sinai Hospital in Milwaukee, and we moved to a duplex on the city's southeast side, convenient to Leon's frozen custard stand as well as weekends in Chicago.

In September 1958, after an extremely difficult delivery, my first son was born with the umbilical cord wound round his neck. It came as no surprise, then, that Tena acted strangely after the delivery. "Postpartum depression," her physician called it. Looking back, I think Tena suffered little bouts of depression almost continuously from the day our first child was born, but I didn't give them the serious consideration they deserved.

Nineteen months later, Tena delivered a second son, and was again diagnosed with postpartum depression. But before the next summer was over, depression had moved on to full-blown mental illness.

Tena couldn't take care of herself, much less care for the children. There were days she left the baby in bed without changing his diaper. Rose, our downstairs neighbor, would stay with Tena or check in on her while I was working, but nothing was being done to help her. Blatantly obvious as her problem might have been to others, I was in denial, and failed to reach out for professional help.

I reached out to no one. I wouldn't share our problem with my family because I didn't want to stress my father, whose health was delicate. It was meaningless to share our problem with Tena's family, for when I spoke of her problems, her mother countered that it was my mental health that was in question. Only my friend Leonard insisted that something be done to help Tena. But finding help would be to no avail, because Tena would convince every physician or psychologist she visited that she didn't have a problem.

At the end of our stay in Milwaukee, I moved my family back to Chicago, where I took a job as administrator of Fox River Pavilion, a facility that was just in the planning stages. It was a new concept in medical treatment — moving those who otherwise would have extended hospital stays to more independent facilities.

We bought a house in Skokie and almost immediately succeeded in finding Tena a psychiatrist. It took her one visit to convince the psychiatrist that she hadn't a problem in the world.

Then came one of the worst days of my life. It was 1966. I came home to a house ransacked from top to bottom, with everything of value gone. There were no pictures on the walls and no clothes in either the children's room or Tena's drawers. There were no children. But my clothes hadn't been disturbed, so I assumed Tena had taken the children with everything else of value to her aunt's house across the street. Without hesitation, I crossed the street and announced that I'd come to pick up my kids.

"You can't have them," came her aunt's reply, to which I responded, "They are my children. They aren't your children, and I want them now. If you want to call the police, call the police. It will be a terrible scene. If you refuse to do this peacefully, I'll knock the door down, walk into the house, and physically take them."

The children came home with me. Needless to say, Tena did not.

The next day, my mother came to care for the children. She stayed the year. Tena filed for divorce. I fought the divorce, but in the end didn't have a choice. Tena demanded the bulk of our assets (which were few) and my new car, but left me half the house. It was not a pleasant situation, I can assure you, but I had the only thing that mattered — full custody of my children.

I was divorced. I was overburdened at work and still upset about the end of my marriage and all that had led up to it. At home, the boys were being taken care of, but they were being spoiled. Spoiled? No, not spoiled. There was no discipline.

After four years at Fox River Pavilion, I had taken a job as administrator at Martha Washington Hospital, a floundering facility of about 50 medical beds plus a 100-year-old alcoholic treatment center. The hospital had been losing money, and in danger of having to close its doors.

I was spending well over 40 hours a week at the hospital and taking care of the boys had turned out to be too much for my mother, so my sister, her husband, and their newly adopted son came to live with us. My sister soon began insisting that I find myself a wife.

ADRIENNE

I met Jack at a "dance" for parents without partners. Maybe he noticed me because I was a wallflower, maybe because I was small. Either way, he asked me to dance and we hit it off immediately. It was obvious to him, and it was obvious to me, that neither of us wanted to be there. I'd come because my friend Margie wanted moral support. Jack had been pushed out of his house by his sister, who was tired of 7-to-11 childcare, and was pressuring Jack to find a wife. I can't say it was love at first sight, because it wasn't, but clearly, something very special happened.

I wouldn't let Jack drive me home. That seemed to bother him, but he evidently got over it, for the very next day he was on the phone, asking me to celebrate St. Patrick's Day with him by going to see Tommy Makem and the Clancy Brothers.

We were married in August of that year. There were 14 of us at the wedding: my parents, Jack's mother, our sisters, my brother and his wife, Jack's brother-in-law, and our four children. We had a couple of thousand dollars between us, two houses, one mortgage, two cars with one being paid out over time, four children aged 2, 4, 8 and 9, and a dog named Cuddles that no one could train.

JACK

After the wedding, my sister and her family moved out, and Adrienne and the girls moved in. I never really gave any thought to where we would live. I just assumed that we would move into my house because it was a much nicer house than Adrienne's. I never thought to ask if she wanted to do that or buy a new house or something else. She never brought up the subject.

It was probably the best move I ever made -- the best thing that ever happened to me. I was very concerned about the welfare of the boys. Adrienne helped them grow into the fine young men they are today.

From time to time, we used to say we should have written a book about putting two families together. From the very beginning, we were one family. We were mother and father to all the kids. I like to believe I treated the girls as my own, and Adrienne treated the boys as her own.

It was a relatively easy adjustment for the girls to make. Adrienne worked with them on understanding the benefits of having two fathers: two fathers to love them, two fathers to bring birthday presents.

It was more difficult for the boys. There were rules, and the rules were enforced. Adrienne refused to make hot pasta for one child and cold pasta for a second child to be served at the same meal. Adrienne took charge of the vitamins, aspirin, and any medications the children might be using, insisting that she'd dispense what was needed when the children needed something. The children's lives were further impacted by the fact that their other parent would take them on weekends. Not every weekend, just some weekends.

ADRIENNE

We had it all. Jack had a big house and I had a little house, so we moved into his big house.

He had boys and I had girls; they became brothers and sisters. He spoke well and I wrote well, so when there was need, we helped each other. Jack even liked to talk, while I liked to listen. That didn't change. Not for a very long time.

In 1968, Jack was administrator of Martha Washington Hospital. He worked long hours. A few months into the marriage we added Mariah — Mr. Mariah when we looked more carefully — the cat who would walk the younger children to school a short six blocks away, and wait in the early afternoon to walk them home.

Under Jack's guidance, the hospital became highly profitable. Jack felt things were going quite well, both for the facility and himself, when he learned that from the beginning, the board president had planned to let him go as soon as the building program was completed. There were words, there was discussion, and there were protests from both staff and physicians demanding that Jack not leave. Circumstances, however, convinced Jack that this was not a board of directors he wanted to work for, and he resigned.

Jack had just resigned when he bumped into Bill Ceas, the man who'd financed Martha Washington Hospital's new building. Ceas had resigned his partnership in the firm he'd been with, and was going to open his own business. Ceas said he'd wanted to talk to Jack about joining him, but felt it inappropriate while Jack was working for his client. Now that Jack was free, Ceas asked if he'd be interested in becoming an investment banker.

Thus in 1971, Jack the hospital administrator became Jack the investment banker, flying around the country, working with small and rural hospitals. Investment banking for Jack was simply an extension of being a hospital administrator. Everything that was vital to running a hospital was important to the development of a sound financing package. Thus, Jack dealt with all the challenges a hospital administrator faces plus the additional burden of providing affordable funding. Jack loved the challenges, and his clients loved him. In a short time, he'd made a name for himself among small and rural hospitals.

There was nothing Jack couldn't do. There was nothing he wouldn't do for a client as long as it was moral, ethical and legal.

I'd never been in the business world per se, and I marveled at the way Jack made all his different projects work for him. I was also impressed at the ease with which he moved from one problem to another, working with boards of directors, community leaders, and politicians until a job was done.

There was no job that went from start to finish without a catastrophe. Papers lost on the day of the closing and the city clerk on vacation. The city clerk found. A project stopped for lack of a legal base. A law enacted. Jack handled the stress of it all like those problems never existed.

Family life always included Tena. Tena would go through bouts of depression, and each time she became depressed, she would sue Jack. She had taken everything of value except the boys, and Jack had even borrowed $1,000 to complete the divorce settlement. Now, she'd call in a rage, wanting to change her visitation dates, but nothing more. No matter how Jack cooperated, she'd take him to court, suing for what he was already willing to give her, forcing him to use what little money we might have had at that moment for legal fees.

Family life hadn't changed when Jack started his new career. He was home less than he had been before, but that was okay. What wasn't okay was that when Jack would fly to a current or potential client to make a presentation, he left the plane exhausted, even if he'd only flown an hour.

Jack had his own personal travel strategy. He preferred to drive to a client if he could, arrive in time to make his presentation, conduct his business, gather his data, and somewhere in the course of all of that, take the client out to dinner. I think it's safe to say that with the possible exception of the children and myself, food was Jack's greatest love. If he had to, he'd spend the night in town and drive home in the morning, but if he wasn't too far from home, he'd turn up some time before dawn.

For flying visits, he developed a slightly different strategy. Since flying made him incredibly tired, he always arranged to arrive a couple of hours before his first appointment, grab a motel, take a nap, and then meet his clients. He actually scheduled visits to allow himself a two-to-three-hour nap before going to a meeting. Arriving at his destination a day ahead of time worked, too.

It seemed strange that Jack was able to drive a long way and arrive relaxed, ready to work, but when he flew to jobs, he arrived tired. I figured he just liked to drive his own car when he could. He'd always loved cars. Otherwise, it didn't make sense and it wasn't important. Correction: it didn't make sense and it didn't **seem** important.

We began to travel together whenever I could arrange to leave the children. Jack was fun to travel with. Any way you look at it, Jack was fun. I tend toward the rigid and compulsive, being an experimental psychologist with tunnel vision. That's great in the laboratory, but rather dull outside.

Jack made my world anything but dull. We explored good food, good theater, old places and new places. A new sight, a new sound, a new artist, a new city -- even a new shopping center made him smile. Happily, it was always his greatest pleasure to share those things with me.

Sometimes, of course, we overindulged. I remember being in Mexico City, having dinner with a Mexican physician friend, when Jack turned a pale greenish yellow, stumbled away from the table, tripped down the two steps leading to the men's room and (I was told) collapsed there in a flood of perspiration.

The diagnosis? "Montezuma's revenge." I remember thinking it would be wise, in the future, to avoid annoying Montezuma.

Back home, I made inquiries. "My husband was taken ill in a restaurant in Mexico City. Do you have any idea what it might have been?"

"Cinnamon," said one. "Cardamom," said another. Poor Jack. I fed him a spoonful of cinnamon one day, and when he didn't go into anaphylactic shock, he got cardamom. I don't remember what all I fed him. I've probably repressed it for the agony I put him through that week — before he collapsed in another restaurant. That was the day I demanded he see Dr. Monte Levinson.

Dr. Levinson, what a man! What a physician! He listened. His nurse drew blood, and he sent us away with instructions to return the following Monday. "And Jack," he said as we headed for the door,

"Adrienne really is stressed with all that you've been through. You know. Not knowing where the anaphylactic shock is coming from. There's a really fine Chinese restaurant that just opened in the neighborhood. Take Adrienne there for dinner Sunday, share a bottle of wine, and I'll see you here on Monday."

So it was that in 1989 Dr. Levinson diagnosed that Jack's problems — from falling asleep on airplanes to going into anaphylactic shock in restaurants — came from a sensitivity to monosodium glutamate.

It was only much later that we learned that it was the MfG in the MSG that was the actual poison, and that many ingredients besides MSG — every flavor enhancer included — contained the same thing and would cause the same reactions.

Treatment? Avoid it. Only later did we learn that meant avoiding MfG.

Jack checked out the ingredients of the Planters Dry Roasted Peanuts that were served on airplanes, and there were those two little words: "monosodium glutamate." Monosodium glutamate all by itself made him tired, while monosodium glutamate with a glass of wine threw him into anaphylactic shock. At least now that he knew what the problem was, he could avoid it. Or so he thought.

There's one truth about sensitivity to MSG that is inescapable. It's really a sensitivity to MfG, and MfG is unavoidable if one eats anything other than fresh, unadulterated, food.

But more than that, find a can of baked beans that you can tolerate, always read the label to be certain that no monosodium glutamate has been added to the ingredients, and when you recover from the world's worst migraine headache and call the people who made the beans you're told that monosodium glutamate had been added to the formula, but the labels on the bean cans had not yet been changed.

Find barbeque ribs made without monosodium glutamate in a restaurant, and the next time you order them the ingredients used to make them will have been changed. As long as Jack could remember, he had enjoyed the barbeque ribs at Carson's restaurant in Skokie, knowing that they were safe for him to eat, never asking about monosodium glutamate in their preparation. Why should he ask about monosodium glutamate? He had eaten there a dozen times or more and not had a problem until he had as bad an attack of anaphylactic shock as I have ever seen. It had not occurred to Jack that Carson's barbeque recipe might change.

ON THE ROAD

Even with four children, we managed to travel. One of our first trips was a driving trip to Florida, visiting Disney World near Orlando and Cape Canaveral.

Around 1974, we took Jack's mother, my parents, the four children and a minivan through Holland, Belgium, and parts of Great Britain. Our oldest son was getting close to college age, the baby was old enough to travel, and we figured it would be the last chance we'd have to travel together.

It was a wonderful vacation, filled with memorable events: the bees at St. Andrews that were attracted to the hairspray on the grandmas' freshly done hairdos; the baby being stung by a wasp during dinner in Scotland; the children mastering the subway in London much better than Jack and I did; the pork kidneys I had for dinner when I, the only French speaker, translated the menu wrong and ordered them for Jack, and the remarkable caves in the middle of nowhere in Belgium, at the end of a seemingly endless drive, worth every bit of the inconvenience of getting there.

In 1979, we made the first of two trips to Hong Kong and China. Going to China with sensitivity to MSG? Not to worry. Piece of cake. What feasts we had! Everything was fresh: rice from the fields, vegetables from the gardens, chickens killed in the yard as we watched. Jack was sensitive to monosodium glutamate. No more, no less. He simply asked that his food be made without monosodium glutamate and everyone was glad to accommodate. In 1979, the Chinese weren't into processed food with flavor enhancers.

In March 1984, friends from Japan came to stay with us in Chicago. June took us to San Francisco. In August, it was a trip to Denver. At the end of the month, we sent the baby off to college.

The first week in December, Jack and I flew to Amsterdam, rented a car and drove to Paris, stopping for dinner at Boyer les Crayeres in Reims. Jack had accumulated enough points with Holiday Inn to give us a free seven-night stay at the Place de la Republic. In truth, the idea of staying at a Holiday Inn in Paris didn't sit well with me. To my surprise and delight, however, our room in the marvelous old building was comfortable and spacious, and the breakfast buffet was sumptuous. To this day I look forward to August, when I can find the fresh figs I first tasted there.

It was another wonderful vacation. We kept to our regular routine: walking and walking, spending time in museums, eating something delicious for lunch (which often included hot chocolate), stopping for a pastry when our feet grew tired, and having a grand dinner at a two-star restaurant. On December 4, we dined at Le Bernardin, December 5 at Duquesnoy, December 6 at Gerard Besson, December 9 at Chez Michel, and December 10 at Trou Gascon.

It was a marvelous time to be in Paris. That December was as mild as December in Paris will ever be. The exchange rate was in our favor, and we bought presents at Baccarat and Lalique, and gloves for ourselves at Muriel. But there was something more, something very special. It was as though Jack had reclaimed his youth. "We'll buy an apartment, buy a car to park at our apartment, and live here. What do you think? We really must do that. There's something in the air here in Paris. Maybe it's like this in all of France. I can't say that I've been feeling poorly. Just getting old. But I feel wonderful here. I haven't felt this well in years."

Of course, we didn't buy the apartment. Not with children still in college and possibly looking at graduate school. But every once in a while I'd hear what turned out to be a recurring refrain: "It was so wonderful in Paris. The air was so good there." There was no thought that MSG-free food made the difference.

In May 1986, we traveled to Japan with my sister. We flew to Tokyo, then took trains, buses, and ferries through much of the country. In Japan, as in Hong Kong and China, a simple request to have food prepared without monosodium glutamate didn't offend anyone. For Jack, there was never a problem.

In September 1987, Jack and I visited Hong Kong, Guangzhou, Guilin, Kunming, Xian, Beijing, Nanjing, Wuxi, Suzhou, and Hangzhou on tour with others. Jack asked for food without monosodium glutamate in it, which was always graciously provided without calling attention to his special request. Evidently, one of the couples on our tour thought Jack was getting something better than the rest of us, and asked if they could have the same meal. Graciously, our hosts brought the meal requested. Not so graciously, the couple sent it back to the kitchen, declaring that it was tasteless.

We visited France again in October 1988, this time with a tour put together by XO Travel Consultants Ltd., called Wine Routes of France. Our guide was a wine merchant who augmented our itinerary with trips to vintners from whom he bought wine. We tasted wine from 10 in the morning till 4 in the afternoon and then, together, had the finest dinners the region had to offer. The people, the wine, the guide, the food, the weather -- nothing could have been better.

Jack's business grew, and now it was his very own business, for he'd left Ceas and Company and opened his own investment banking firm. With his own business came greater responsibility and, I suppose, greater pressure. Then, with the passage of time, came signs of aging. Short temper here, short temper there. Jack could be tired, cranky, argumentative and verbally abusive. He didn't have as much energy or stamina as he used to, and he had an aching bone or two. "Blood pressure a bit too high," said the doctor. "Time to take off some weight."

Hindsight, they say, is 20/20. If Jack or I had stopped to think about it, would we have realized that when traveling outside the country, Jack always felt better than he did at home?

Chapter Six

On the Art of Deceiving the Public

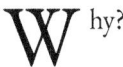hy?

Why does the FDA allow the intentional addition of neurotoxic processed free glutamic acid (MfG) to processed food?

Why aren't consumers aware of MfG's toxic potential?

Why aren't healthcare professionals aware of the fact that obesity, reproductive disorders and retinal degeneration can be caused or exacerbated through the use of MfG?

Why aren't healthcare professionals alert to the symptoms of MfG toxicity?

Why? Because Ajinomoto has made sure that things happened that way.

1: Start with a Well-Funded Organization.
History tells us that in 1969, the International Glutamate Technical Committee (IGTC) was founded as an association of companies engaged in the manufacture, sale and commercial use of glutamates. It sponsored, gathered, and disseminated research on the use and safety of monosodium glutamate; designed and implemented research protocols and provided financial assistance to researchers; promoted acceptance of monosodium glutamate as a food ingredient, and represented members'

collective interests[97]. Those collective interests were to sell monosodium glutamate. It would appear that the IGTC was the brainchild of Ajinomoto Co., a leading manufacturer of monosodium glutamate. But I often wonder if it wasn't Andrew Ebert who thought up the whole thing. Ebert had been with Minnesota Mining and Minerals when they were producing MSG.

It was reported in 1994 that the IGTC was an association composed of physicians and/or scientists either employed by producers or users of glutamic acid and its salts, or doing research on it in university laboratories. Its annual budget was $250,000. Membership was $2,000/year[98]. A former IGTC member told us Ajinomoto made up any shortfall between member-provided funds and that quarter-million.

In 1977, the IGTC spun off The Glutamate Association, with both organizations having close ties to the Robert H. Kellen Company of Atlanta, Ga. and Washington, DC. Kellen is a trade organization and association management firm that specializes in the food, pharmaceutical, and healthcare industries. Richard (Rich) Cristol, executive director of The Glutamate Association, was also vice president of The Kellen Company; and in 1992, Andrew (Andy) Ebert, Ph.D., chairman of the IGTC, was also senior vice president of The Kellen Company[99,100].

Membership in The Glutamate Association has always been secret. In the early 1990s, however, a member friend told us that Ajinomoto, Archer Daniels Midland, Campbell, Corn Products Corporation, McCormick & Company, Nestle, Pfizer Laboratories, and Takeda were among its members.

2: Identify and Employ MDs and PhDs to conduct research designed by your organization to fail to find any negative effects of MSG, and to speak publicly about the safety of your product.

Once established, the IGTC assembled a cadre of scientists and others who conducted research for them and/or spoke publicly about the safety of monosodium glutamate. In the 1970s and 1980s, research sponsors were acknowledged.

The names of researchers Altman, Anantharaman, Auer, Bunyan, Ebert, Fernstrom, Filer, Garattini, Geha, Germano, Giacometti, Goldschmiedt, Heywood, Iwata, Kelly, Kenney, Kerr, Matsuzawa,

Morselli, Newman, Owen, Patterson, Pulce, Reynolds, Saxon, Schiffman, Simon, Stegink, Stevenson, Takasaki, Tarasoff, Williams, Woessner, and Yang have been notable, although there have been others. In the late 1990s we saw the names Torii, Shi, Jinap and Hajeb added to the roster.

Steve Taylor deserves special mention. Although a prominent representative of the glutamate industry, he's not included with the others because his ties to the IGTC have not openly been acknowledged. Although Taylor has repeatedly spoken out about the safety of MSG[101], only once to our knowledge has he acknowledged his ties to the IGTC.

Taylor has done little or no basic research related to monosodium glutamate safety/toxicity, but is respected for his knowledge about food allergy. He has served as an officer of the Toxicology and Safety Evaluation Division and a member of the Expert Panel on Food Safety and Nutrition of the IFT[102]. His name appears prominently on advisory boards such as the Food Allergy Network[103], and editorial boards such as the *Encyclopedia of Food Science Food Technology and Nutrition*[104]. When he introduces himself, he typically refers to his University of Nebraska affiliation, but not to the fact that he's an agent of The Glutamate Association, the IGTC, and/or Ajinomoto[105,106].

A number of years ago, Taylor appeared with Jack on a small market television program in Chicago, discussing MSG. That was the only time we heard him admit to being a spokesperson for the glutamate industry. Jack always chuckled when he recalled how Taylor bolted from the studio after the show, possibly because he hadn't been able to enhance the image of monosodium glutamate, or maybe because toward the end of the show, the moderator had asked him if he wanted Jack dead.

The focus of researchers who represent the glutamate industry has always been to demonstrate that use of monosodium glutamate is "safe." The early research of both Richard Kenney and Roland Auer had suggested that glutamic acid might have toxic potential[107,108] while their subsequent studies and/or public statements proclaimed that MSG is safe[109,110]. We found it interesting that their change in focus coincided with research support provided by the glutamate industry.

By and large, those who've represented the glutamate industry have produced research relative to the safety of monosodium glutamate only in response to encouragement from the glutamate industry. Moreover, although the first challenges to the safety of monosodium glutamate were based on brain lesions and subsequent neuroendocrine disorders, only two glutamate industry representatives, Richard J. Wurtman, M.D. and Roland Auer, M.D., Ph.D. have been neuroscientists.

Until he was mentioned to the FDA as having been responsible for supplying placebos containing excitotoxic aspartic acid (in aspartame) to the researchers conducting glutamate-safety double-blind studies for him, Ebert had been key to the research operations of the IGTC. This professionally respected pharmacologist and toxicologist had been with the IGTC from the beginning, recruiting researchers to carry out the research designed for them. In each case, that research has enabled Ebert's people to proclaim (without justification) that a new study has demonstrated that monosodium glutamate is a harmless food additive.

Ebert is the personification of the IGTC, and his influence can be felt at every level. He's served on the FDA Food Advisory Committee; the Grocery Manufacturers of America (Technical Committee on Food Protection, the Codex Subcommittee on Food Additives and the GRAS-FASEB Monograph Committee); the National Food Processors Association; the Institute of Food Technologists (Technology Toxicology and Safety Evaluation Division, and Scientific Lecturer); the National Research Council of the National Academy of Sciences Assembly of Life Sciences (Food and Nutrition Board: the Committee on Food Protection, and the GRAS List Survey); the AMA (Industry Liaison Panel); the FAO/WHO Codex Alimentarius Food Standards Program as an industry observer; and the International Food Additives Council as executive director[111].

As a food industry pharmacologist and toxicologist, Ebert has provided scientific and technical expertise for programs of many associations managed by The Kellen Company.

Ebert has also been an active member of the IFT, but he's not the only IFT glutamate-industry spokesperson. Daryl Altman, M.D., worked for former IFT president Al Clausi, vice chairman of Allerx, Inc. and its medical affiliate, The Food Allergy Center. Dr. Altman often speaks, or has spoken publicly about the safety of monosodium glutamate, often with Steve Taylor. The IFIC has promoted them as speakers without mentioning the fact that they represented the glutamate industry. L.T. Chiaramonte, M.D., who has co-authored work for the IGTC with

Altman, has served on the medical advisory board of The Food Allergy Center.

It appears that since his exposure, Ebert no longer sits as chairman of the IGTC.

In 2009, we came across his name as being on the IGTC Executive Committee[112], but have seen little more about him since then. His move from the glutamate industry limelight coincided with our posting information on our website about his role in designing the IGTC's "scientific" studies and supplying aspartame-laced placebos (placebos that cause reactions similar, if not identical, to those caused by MSG) to his researchers. Toward the end of the 1990s, we began to see the names of Takeshi Kimura and Yoshi-hisa Sugita, Ph.D., associated with the IGTC[113]. I wonder if that was a policy change for Ajinomoto, or if Americans were no longer willing to take over as IGTC chairman. Both Kimura and Sugita came straight from Ajinomoto[114,115].

Jumping ahead to 2022, it looked like the IGTC had moved its offices to Brussels, with Michael Rogers, IGTC chairman, leaving The Glutamate Association and its International Glutamate Information Service (IGIS) to run Ajinomoto's U.S. operation while the IGTC continues to focus on whatever it will take (no holds barred) to keep MSG profitable. The IGTC's aims are to "study, assemble and disseminate scientific data and information related to all aspects of the safety, quality and use of glutamate and its salts, particularly monosodium glutamate with a particular emphasis on their use in foods for human beings" and "promote the uses of glutamates as food ingredients especially on an international level." The six organizations that carry out its work are:

EUROPE — PARIS:
European Committee for Umami (ECU)
JAPAN — TOKYO — SOUTH KOREA — SEOUL:
Amino Acids Seasoning Alliance of Northeast Asia (ASANA)
REPUBLIC OF CHINA — TAIPEI:
Taiwan Amino Acid Manufacturers Association ROC (TAAMA)
SOUTH AMERICA — SAO PAULO:
Institute for Glutamate Sciences in South America (IGSSA)
SOUTHEAST ASIA — BANGKOK:
Regional Committee for Glutamate Sciences (RCGS)

U.S.A. — WASHINGTON, DC:
The Glutamate Association United States (TGA)

I Googled Ebert just to see what he'd been doing, and at the time came across a bio that listed him as a consultant to The Kellen Company (which shares offices with the IGTC), but failed to mention any association with the IGTC. I also found that he headed his own consulting firm (EMT, Inc.) and was still active in groups such as the U.S. Pharmacopeia (USP), where in 2010 he served as chair of the Food Ingredients Expert Committee[116]. According to the USP website as it appeared on June 29, 2010:

> "The United States Pharmacopeia (USP) is a non-governmental, official public standards-setting authority for prescription and over-the-counter medicines and other healthcare products manufactured or sold in the United States. USP also sets widely recognized standards for food ingredients and dietary supplements. USP sets standards for the quality, purity, strength, and consistency of these products–critical to the public health. USP's standards are recognized and used in more than 130 countries around the globe. These standards have helped to ensure public health throughout the world for close to 200 years"[117].

In 2010, we saw Ebert on YouTube speaking as chair of USP's Food Ingredients Expert Committee, discussing the seventh edition of the Food Chemicals Codex and the importance of quality ingredient standards in food safety[118]. Somehow, I don't think Ebert is suggesting to these people that monosodium glutamate has toxic potential.

Ebert has worn, and may still wear, so many different hats at one time, that when he presents information to any person or organization, he can point to his affiliation with a neutral organization while failing to mention an affiliation with an organization that his audience might find inappropriate or offensive. The importance of this attribute was driven home when we saw FDA Commissioner David Kessler's letter to Ebert of the Kellen Corporation, inviting him to be a member of the FDA

Food Advisory Committee. His nomination to that advisory committee didn't refer to his affiliation with the IGTC, but listed him only as senior vice president of The Kellen Company. His acceptance was written on The Kellen Company letterhead[118].

Ronald Simon, M.D. and Donald D. Stevenson, M.D. of Scripps Clinic and Research Foundation, La Jolla, Calif., have vigorously represented the glutamate industry since 1995. In 1991, Simon, with Dean D. Metcalfe, M.D. and Hugh R. Sampson, M.D., had praised the work of David Allen, M.D., who'd found that MSG can act as an asthma trigger. In fact, Simon, Metcalfe, and Sampson had included Allen's study in their book, *Food Allergy: Adverse Reactions to Foods and Food Additives*[119]. In a letter to Dr. George Schwartz, that Schwartz shared with Jack, Allen wrote, "Last week my friend Ron Simon from the Scripps Clinic called me and asked me to participate in a symposium at the American Academy of Allergy meeting in San Francisco in March of next year. I'll be speaking on sulfites and MSG and their potential to provoke asthma"[120].

On August 31, 1995, the FDA released a report on the safety of monosodium glutamate in food, done by FASEB[93]. In that report, FASEB acknowledged that monosodium glutamate was an asthma trigger, and that MSG doses as low as half-a-gram had triggered monosodium glutamate reactions. On the day before that report was to be released, Simon and Stevenson wrote to inform the FDA that they believed FASEB had made a grave error in stating that monosodium glutamate was known to be an asthma trigger, for they had found Allen's work to be lacking[121]. In 1995, Simon and Stevenson were engaged in research funded by the IGTC[122].

We found it most interesting that Simon and Stevenson knew what was in the FASEB report before it was released. We were reminded that in 1994, glutamate industry friend and *Food and Chemical Toxicology* editor Joseph Borzelleca had known that the 1994 "final draft" of that same FASEB report would be rejected by the FDA and returned to FASEB for "clarification."

I'm inclined to tell you more about the work of Simon and Stevenson because they have so conscientiously represented the glutamate industry. In 1996, the newsletter of the NOMSG consumer group reported that when a monosodium glutamate-sensitive person responded to an advertisement in the Los Angeles Times for test subjects for a Scripps Clinic study, she was told that "1) If she feared her asthma reactions to be serious that she should not apply for the study; 2) that the person who was screening the applicants didn't believe that monosodium glutamate could cause asthma reactions; and 3) that this particular person was most likely responding to sulfites, and not to monosodium glutamate"[123]. By this and other methods, persons who were sensitive to monosodium glutamate were eliminated from participation in Scripps Clinic studies of adverse reactions to monosodium glutamate.

On May 24, 1997, I wrote to Simon, asking him about work he and Stevenson might be doing for Ajinomoto or one of its agents, on the general subject of sensitivity to MSG[124].

In a May 28, 1997 letter, Simon responded, saying, "There is no study that we are doing for Ajinomoto or one of their agents, on the general subjective sensitivity to MSG. The abstract presented at the February 1997 American Academy of Allergy Asthma & Immunology (AAAAI) meetings was a preliminary report of an ongoing study we designed concerning MSG sensitivity in asthmatics"[125].

Quite to the contrary, however, the program for that AAAAI meeting included an abstract for a poster session, "The Role of Monosodium L-Glutamate (MSG) in Asthma: Does it Exist?" by Stevenson et al. funded by the IGTC[122].

Others who stand out as loyal agents of Ajinomoto and its IGTC are Lloyd Filer and Lewis Stegink from the University of Iowa, and their co-author W. Ann Reynolds, formerly at the University of Illinois. They, along with Richard Kenney and Richard Wurtman, not only produced IGTC-approved studies and participated in their workshops, but spoke out repeatedly about the safety of monosodium glutamate. Their work demonstrates both the glutamate industry's power and the willingness of reputable researchers, and medical facilities to cooperate in industry's efforts to convince both health professionals and consumers that MSG is safe.

3: Use a Variety of Strategies, Changing them From Time to Time.

When focusing on the safety of monosodium glutamate and the other ingredients that contain MfG, the Glutes continue to use five fairly distinct creative strategies.

First, there's research that claims to have demonstrated that the product, monosodium glutamate, is safe. More precisely, the claim associated with any single piece of research is that the study failed to produce any evidence that monosodium glutamate causes asthma or Chinese restaurant syndrome. All that glutamate industry researchers have to do to accomplish their goal is to look at the wrong thing, at the wrong time, in people who aren't sensitive to MfG, and for good measure, lace placebos used in double-blind studies with aspartame. The propaganda people can then spin the story until it reads that monosodium glutamate is safe.

Second, there's suppression of information. When contradictory or embarrassing information has been published in books or journals, those in positions of power block media coverage. When criticism of glutamate industry research is offered for publication, editors refuse to publish those critiques. When criticism of deceptive and misleading research reports is anticipated, researchers publish in journals that don't accept comment following publication.

Third is the dissemination of deceptive and/or misleading information. In the privacy of our own home, Jack and I sometimes referred to these as lies. Some are trivial. Some are not. All are designed to sell product. "Monosodium glutamate has been in use for over 2,000 years" is a statement you'll now rarely see, since we pointed out that monosodium glutamate was invented in 1908[8]. If you realize that asthma, migraine headaches, depression, and seizures are known to be triggered by MfG, the statement, "The reactions to monosodium glutamate are mild and transitory" takes on the characteristics of a bold-faced lie.

Fourth is the component we called "dirty tricks." We thought of these as activities aimed at a particular person. Canceling airplane and hotel reservations we had made for attendance at a conference might be called a dirty trick. Interrupting service on our fax machine might be another.

Fifth is the glutamate industry's skill in marketing in general, and in lobbying both appointed and elected officials to follow its lead in proclaiming monosodium glutamate to be safe. The FDA, the National Institutes of Health (NIH), the EPA, the USDA, and the California Department of Pesticide Regulation are among those that appear to have been successfully lobbied.

4: Change the Rules of the Game as Needed.

Over the years, while their mission to sell monosodium glutamate has remained the same, the glutamate industry's game plan has changed. In 1969, following Olney's demonstration that monosodium glutamate killed brain cells in the area of the arcuate nucleus of the hypothalamus, the glutamate industry sponsored animal studies that claimed to replicate the work of Olney and others, but did not do so[6]. In the series of industry-sponsored studies that claimed to have found no damage caused by monosodium glutamate, researchers used animal subjects that differed from Olney's, waited to examine brain tissue until all traces of brain damage would have disappeared, offered analyses of brain tissue in areas outside of the arcuate nucleus, and used inappropriate methods for staining and examining brain tissue.

By the late 1970s, the neurotoxic effects of monosodium glutamate were undeniable. Neuroscientists were actually using monosodium glutamate as an ablative or provocative tool with which to selectively kill brain cells in order to study brain function and promote drug development[126,127]. Undaunted, those in the glutamate industry simply began to claim that animal research didn't speak to the toxicity of monosodium glutamate because research done on animals doesn't represent the human condition. The FDA never blinked an eye.

Glutamate industry-sponsored human studies began in 1970 with work done by Morselli and Garattini[128] and Bazzano, D'Elia, and Olson[129] that appears to have been done in response to 1968 letters written to the *New England Journal of Medicine* discussing the reactions experienced by Dr. Ho Man Kwok following meals taken in a restaurant serving northern Chinese food. They and other glutamate industry researchers produced studies which, they said, demonstrated that monosodium glutamate didn't cause adverse reactions. Some were double-blind studies that used placebos containing excitotoxic (brain damaging) aspartic acid (found in aspartame). All were flawed to the point of being fraudulent. All were studies on which the glutamate industry bases its assertion that MfG is safe for human consumption. All are studies that the FDA has refused to challenge.

Early in the 21st century we anticipated that in the not-too-distant future, Ajinomoto would choose to direct attention away from its badly flawed human double-blind studies. No longer would the glutamate industry focus on the claim that essentially no one is sensitive to MSG, the acronym MSG being understood at the time to stand for all free glutamic acid (MfG). Instead, Ajinomoto and friends would agree to label MfG, and say that in so doing, they would prove that people who say they are sensitive to MSG are really not sensitive to MSG.

Ajinomoto had been laying the foundation for implementing this change in game plan for years, with full cooperation from the FDA. In fact, the last play was put into effect when the Glutes had the FDA reject the draft of what has since become the "independent" 1995 FASEB report on the safety of MSG, requiring that the FDA include justification for identifying MfG only when there was more than 3 grams MfG in an ingredient.

The strategy would be to advertise that the MfG in processed food would be labeled, without mentioning the fact that some MfG, but not all MfG, would be identified on product labels. The plan called for identification of MfG in processed food only if the amount of MfG in a given ingredient was greater than 3 grams. And few, if any ingredients contain as much as 3 grams of MfG.

From what we know about the content of MfG in processed food, we'd estimate that by labeling products that contained 3 grams or more MfG per serving, approximately 99 percent of the MfG in processed food would remain unidentified. The excessive amounts of MfG consumed in processed foods are due to the fact that a processed or ultra-processed food contains more than one MfG-containing ingredient, and more than one processed or ultra-processed food is eaten at a time. Moreover, virtually every ingredient in processed foods contains MfG. (See Chapter 9 for additional information).

Evidence of the FDA's cooperation in this endeavor will be found in FASEB's published Analysis of Adverse Reactions to Monosodium Glutamate (MSG)[93] and in the FDA's 1996 Advance Notice of Proposed Rulemaking[130].

Chapter Seven

Fraud by Any Other Name Can't Be Prosecuted

L ong before we thought of looking to medical literature for information about MSG, Olney and others had proved beyond the shadow of a doubt that monosodium glutamate fed to young laboratory animals kills brain cells in the arcuate nucleus of the hypothalamus, a brain region that helps control endocrine function. In addition, Olney and others had demonstrated that monosodium glutamate fed to young laboratory animals subsequently caused behavior and endocrine disorders such as stunted growth, ADHD, obesity, and reproductive disorders[131-139].

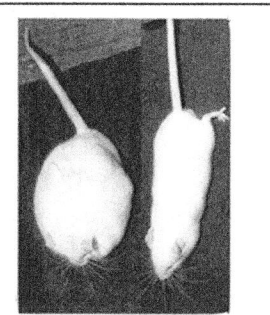

(Fig. 3. A 9-month-old Swiss albino mouse (left) that was treated, as a newborn, with [monosodium glutamate] is shown beside the heaviest untreated male (right) from the same litter[140]. Reproduced with permission of the author.)

In the 1970s, 1980s, and early 1990s, cooperation between individual researchers, universities and/or medical schools, government, and industry was openly acknowledged. When a study was published, a note told who sponsored the study. Thus, it was clearly stated that studies of monosodium glutamate safety from the University of Iowa College of Medicine and the University of Illinois Medical Center (where W. Ann Reynolds was then on faculty) were financed and/or orchestrated by Ajinomoto, Gerber Products Company, G.D. Searle & Company (inventor of aspartame), the IGTC, and Searle Laboratories. Funding also came from various institutes of the NIH.

The University of Iowa College of Medicine has a long history of cooperation with food and drug industry interests. In 1967, the Mead-Johnson Professorship in the Department of Pediatrics was established by the Mead-Johnson and Company Foundation, Inc., and Filer moved from Mead-Johnson (a producer of infant formula) to the University of Iowa College of Medicine, where he served as Mead-Johnson Professor from 1967 through 1977[147]. Filer remained a spokesman for the glutamate industry until his death[148].

The allegiance of these people to the glutamate industry has been remarkable. In 1970, Filer chaired the National Academy of Sciences (NAS) subcommittee on Safety and Suitability of MSG and Other Substances in Baby Food, which issued the report, "Safety and Suitability of Monosodium Glutamate for Use in Baby Food"[149]. At the time, the FDA was using the NAS to do its studies, much as it later used FASEB. Notwithstanding the fact that Olney had demonstrated that glutamic acid caused brain lesions and neuroendocrine disorders in laboratory animals, with infant animals being most at risk, Filer's subcommittee concluded, without reference to data, that glutamate was safe[149].

Subsequently, the NAS committee was criticized. Most of its members were found to have close financial ties to the food industry. Chairman Filer, then Mead-Johnson Professor at the University of Iowa, was found to be receiving money from both the baby food and glutamate industries[150].

Toward the end of the 1990s, I began to summarize the glutamate industry-sponsored human studies[8]. Although they were carried out by a variety of researchers at a variety of medical schools and universities, the essential elements of each study were the same. It was clear to me that the goal of each was to produce a study that failed to find a relationship between ingestion of monosodium glutamate and production of adverse reactions.

Step one would be to impress the reader with a sophisticated sounding "randomized, double-blind, placebo-controlled, multiple-challenge crossover design study," or something equally dazzling. Random selection of subjects is essential in studies that are to be generalized to the population from which subjects are drawn. But subjects in these studies were not randomly drawn. Subjects were always volunteers who claimed to be sensitive to monosodium glutamate, and there is nothing random about that. The only thing that was random was the order in which subjects receive the monosodium glutamate test material as opposed to the placebo. Consequently, not one of these industry-sponsored studies met the assumptions of the statistical tests used. So even if there were no other flaws in these studies, having failed to meet the assumptions on which the statistical tests were built, the IGTC-sponsored studies were meaningless.

As you might suspect, the studies had other flaws. It was claimed that subjects serving in these studies were self-selected MSG-sensitive people, but they were often students who were offered several hundred dollars to participate in a study (sometimes for just a couple of hours) only if they said they were sensitive to MSG. Might not a graduate student be tempted to claim MSG sensitivity if the reward for spending a few hours in an office would be several hundred dollars? No one verified that subjects were actually sensitive to MSG.

How did we know such things? Our daughter was a student on the Chicago campus of Northwestern University, where one of the studies was being conducted. There were flyers asking for subjects to participate in an MSG study hanging on bulletin boards everywhere, and she inquired. She thought we might be interested.

Soliciting informed consent is a requirement of human research done in all universities and medical schools. Informed consent means subjects have been told what the study will entail, and agree to participate. In so doing, prospective subjects are given some indication of what the test is all about, and the procedures to which they'll be subjected. Do you think MSG-sensitive people would line up to join a study where they knew they were going to be fed monosodium glutamate? I wouldn't.

Most flaws won't be obvious. For example, IGTC researchers counted reactions only if they occurred within two hours following ingestion of monosodium glutamate, even though reactions to monosodium glutamate occur anywhere from immediately following ingestion to as much as 48 hours later. For years, the glutamate industry has broadcast the story that reactions to monosodium glutamate are mild and transitory, occurring (**only** occurring is the inference) between 10 minutes and an hour after ingestion. Neither the man on the street nor his physician would have any idea that the time allowed for collecting responses in these studies was inappropriate.

Headache, vomiting and nausea, diarrhea, abdominal pain and cramps, and change in mood quality or level represented 42 percent of the reactions reported to the FDA when its Adverse Reaction Monitoring System was compiling a list of reactions to MSG. Most of the industry-sponsored studies ignored those reactions, counting only numbness, tingling, and tightness associated with Chinese restaurant syndrome as recordable reactions.

The assertion that "a subject who reacts to placebo material as well as to monosodium glutamate test material is not sensitive to monosodium glutamate" is one of the fundamental fictions on which marketing monosodium glutamate as "safe" is built.

Think about it for a moment. Imagine that on one day a person is given a piece of licorice and breaks out in hives, and on another day the same person is given a piece of chocolate and breaks out in hives. Is the fact that a person given chocolate breaks out in hives evidence that licorice doesn't cause that person to similarly break out in hives? Of course not. But the glutamate industry claims that people who get migraine headaches after eating MSG aren't sensitive to it, because they also get migraines from ingesting some form of MfG and/or aspartame in something they call a "placebo." The IGTC actually set up a series of double-blind studies wherein subjects were given MfG in monosodium glutamate as test material and MfG-containing autolyzed yeast, hydrolyzed protein, and/or citric acid as well as aspartame in placebos. The glutamate industry has always been so incredibly powerful within the FDA and the medical community that its creative (and misleading) research designs go unchallenged.

According to Ebert, the use of aspartame in placebos began in 1978,[29] which was well before 1983 when aspartame was approved by the FDA for use in beverages.

Over and above the fact that use of aspartame in placebos is grossly inappropriate, the fact that once approved for use, aspartame-containing products were supposed to carry a warning on their labels didn't deter the glutamate industry from using the substance or the FDA from allowing its use. Aspartame contains phenylalanine (which adversely affects one in 15,000 Americans), aspartic acid (an excitatory amino acid) and a methyl ester. Aspartic acid and glutamic acid load on the same receptors in the brain cause the same brain damage and neuroendocrine disorders in experimental animals, and, with the exception of blindness related to aspartame ingestion, cause virtually the same adverse reactions in humans.

There were more than 7,000 unsolicited reports of adverse reactions to aspartame filed with the FDA before the list was closed. It should surprise no one, therefore, that glutamate industry researchers find as many reactions following ingestion of an aspartame-containing placebo as they find following ingestion of monosodium glutamate test material.

By the time I'd completed my research, having reviewed all the IGTC-sponsored studies, I understood just how the IGTC produced study after study that found no association between ingestion of monosodium glutamate and adverse reactions. I'd observed that while a variety of researchers worked on the various studies, and the work was produced at different universities and medical schools, the designs of each study were essentially the same. Only the details varied. While the flaws of each study could be dismissed as shoddy science, sloppy scholarship, or inadvertent error, taking the group of studies as a whole, it appeared that there was clear intent to deceive the public about the safety of monosodium glutamate.

Intent to deceive? Could it be otherwise? Given the methodological flaws inherent in their work, and their unwillingness to change their protocols after those flaws were pointed out to them, we were drawn to the notion that it was with intent that IGTC researchers moved from a predetermined conclusion (that their product is "safe") to design and implementation of research guaranteed to bring readers back to that predetermined conclusion.

And they brought their study protocols to the FDA, where they were approved.

Jack and I discussed the fact that there are some circles where deception with intent to deceive is defined as fraud. But with the FDA on their team, and without a whistleblower, there would seem to be no way to prove beyond a reasonable doubt that all of the flaws in glutamate industry research design and implementations are due to anything more than stupidity, ineptness, and/or sloppy research. We had already learned through painful experience that industry's power extends into the courts, and thus we decided it would be an exercise in futility to begin a discussion about glutamate industry fraud. So, we didn't.

For those who'd like an example of the glutamate industry-sponsored human studies, I recommend the one done by Tarasoff and Kelly of the Department of Chemistry, Faculty of Business & Technology, University of Western Sydney, Campbelltown, NSW, Australia[72]. I suggest it because my critique of the study was published (after a year's dispute with the publisher and journal editors) and is readily available[73].

The contents of the placebos, which were identified in the eventually published study, were noted only as "powdered beverage packets from the sponsor." Neither the use of aspartame nor a change in placebo ingredients is mentioned in the published study. The study, which was initiated in 1992, was published in 2000.

In 1990, I questioned research done by Markus Goldschmiedt, J.S. Redfern, and Mark Feldman[154] that used beef broth as a placebo for controls. In the U.S. you can't purchase commercially prepared beef broth that doesn't contain MfG (hydrolyzed protein, yeast extract, textured vegetable protein, flavoring, etc.). I questioned the possible unwitting bias in placebo material in a letter to the editor of the *American Journal of Clinical Nutrition*. The letter wasn't published and no informative reply was received. I questioned Feldman about the contents of the placebo. He replied that he didn't know the content of the various materials he used.

It had become clear the glutamate industry was having its way, and the fact that the food additive monosodium glutamate caused brain lesions and endocrine disorders was being universally ignored. We'd tried to point out that it was really quite obvious that the endocrine systems of the unborn and the very young were being damaged by MfG fed to infants in utero through their mothers' diets; by MfG ingested by nursing mothers and passed on to infants through their milk; by the MfG in infant formula (loaded with hydrolyzed proteins and other sources of MfG), and by the MSG and MfG in vaccines that would be mainlined to infants. But the glutamate industry has done its job so well, that information stemming from the animal studies was, and still is, given no consideration.

Even the obvious role played by endocrine-disrupting MfG in the obesity epidemic, was being ignored. In early 2022, I attempted to publish evidence demonstrating that quantities of MfG ingested by pregnant women cause damage to the brains of fetuses followed by intransigent obesity, just as MfG fed to neonatal animals causes brain damage to the arcuate nuclei of those neonatal animals -- brain damage that is followed by gross obesity. Those submissions were denied publication by *Obesity*, the journal of The Obesity Society. One of the reasons cited for rejection was what that the article was by a single author.

Finally, we observed that when data don't support certain predetermined conclusions, researchers may draw conclusions that don't follow from the results of their studies. Moreover, if a glutamate industry-sponsored study doesn't work out as desired, it might simply not be published. A study undertaken at the Medical College of Virginia by Donald Kirby, M.D. is an example of such "buried" research[155].

Chapter Eight

When More Than Rigged Research Is Needed

C onsumer pressure to expose the toxic potential of MSG/MfG continued; the growing science on neurodegenerative disease continued to implicate glutamic acid; a growing number of diverse disease conditions were being linked to the glutamate cascade; and members of the U.S. Congress were privately admitting that they, personally, were sensitive to MSG. But industry-inspired articles attesting to the safety of MSG continued to be published by agents of the glutamate industry, and continued to receive coverage in the press while almost anything that might have suggested MSG has toxic potential was ignored.

Ajinomoto and its IGTC continued maintaining that their product, monosodium glutamate, posed no threat to humans. But what about those who had different opinions?

John Olney was one who had a different opinion. He had published research to that effect in peer-reviewed journals throughout the 1970s[22]. In 1972, he testified before the Senate Select Committee on Nutrition and Human Needs that ingestion of MSG places humans at risk, with the greatest risk being for the very young. What happened to that information?

We learned about suppression of information firsthand when food editors of major newspapers with whom I'd established good relations refused to talk to me. We learned more when an article that was supposed to cover a talk given by Dr. Russell Blaylock at the 1994 NOMSG convention in Chicago, focused instead on the wonders of monosodium glutamate[77]. Mention of MSG by major media sources has been virtually nonexistent since *60 Minutes* aired its story about MSG's toxic effects in 1991. Sometime after that aired, Nancy Millman, writing as a freelance writer for the *Chicago Sun Times*, did an article focusing on Jack's activities and his efforts to have MSG labeled. According to Millman, prior to beginning her work, she'd cleared the story with her editor—but the article was never published.

Similarly, the *Baltimore Sun* accepted and then refused to print an article on MSG written by Linda Bonvie, and an editor at the *New York Times* told Bonvie she wouldn't take a story that even mentioned MSG. According to Bonvie, the editor said she was unwilling to face the pressure she knew would come from running such a piece. In 1991, Don Hewett of *60 Minutes* said, on television, that he'd never had so much pressure applied to him by industry as he had prior to the airing of the MSG segment. Although rated by *TV Guide* as one of the two most watched *60 Minutes* segments of 1991, to this day *60 Minutes* hasn't touched on the subject again, and when asked, refused to do so.

Since 1991, the media have had little to say about MSG other than that food containing it is safe to consume. The only coverage of a lawsuit we filed against the FDA for failure to require appropriate labeling of MSG was carried by CNN, CBN, and the *St. Louis Post Dispatch* when the suit was filed, and by CBN and the *St. Louis Post Dispatch* when the court's decision was handed down.

In 1998, the *Washington Post* carried an article about monosodium glutamate by Robert L. Wolke[156] that might as well have come directly from The Glutamate Association. Following its publication, I wrote to the *Post* editor, detailing the bias in Wolke's article, and several days later, found the following message from the Post's Fanny Zollicoffer on my answering machine:

> about your "...letter to the editor about MSG, and the article we had in the food section. We'd like to publish your letter. It's being considered for the free fall page on Saturday. And I'm just calling to confirm that you wrote the letter and put your name on it and sent it to no other newspaper."

When I called several days later to inquire why my letter hadn't appeared in the paper, I was told the editors had decided not to print it.

There are other ways information can be suppressed. The glutamate industry suppresses information by drawing attention away from the truth and focusing, instead, on the trivial or untrue. Critics of the industry are disparaged or made the subject of jokes. (Critics don't report adverse reactions, they "complain.") Irrelevant information is given in response to serious questions about the safety of a product. ("If you eat too much of anything, you'll get sick.") Falsehoods are recited by alleged authorities. ("A blood-brain barrier prevents amino acids you eat from entering the brain.")

Existing data may be distorted or trivialized. Every report of human suffering is labeled anecdotal and dismissed. Research misconduct, if detected, is excused as an error of judgment or sloppy work. The industry's suppression of information, in all its many forms, is ignored by anyone with the authority to do anything about it. Finally, those in positions of power to do otherwise, ignore the fact that quantities of badly flawed research and repeated instances of direct suppression of information have contributed to the acceptance of monosodium glutamate as a harmless food additive. In America, information, including data, can be suppressed without accountability.

When there's no getting around the fact that MSG causes adverse reactions, as is the case with migraine headaches, the glutamate industry and its colleagues at the FDA simply don't discuss those reactions. The FASEB, in a report done for the FDA and published in July 1995[93] covered the subject of asthma in some detail, but virtually ignored the subject of migraine headaches, despite the fact that 43 percent of the reactions reported to the FDA's Adverse Reactions Monitoring System by MSG-sensitive people (before the FDA stopped compiling reports of adverse reactions to MSG) were migraine headaches[157].

Ignoring criticism is actually a fundamental strategy of the Glutes and their friends at the FDA. When the FDA was informed that the placebos in industry's MSG-safety studies contained material that would cause reactions identical to those caused by MSG, the FDA ignored the information. Similarly, the Citizen Petition filed in 2021 requesting that MSG and MfG be stripped of their GRAS status is being ignored.

Suppression of information implies there's information in existence that isn't communicated. Slightly different is the FDA policy of suppressing information by not providing it in the first place, i.e., not alerting people to things they might benefit from knowing. At one time, when consumers were relatively vocal about their sensitivities to MSG and aspartame, the FDA found it prudent to demonstrate that "they were studying the matter," and keep records of reports from consumers who wrote that they'd experienced adverse reactions to MSG and/or aspartame. But the FDA didn't solicit reports from consumers. Neither did it announce, in any source commonly accessed by consumers, that such reports were being collected. It was only through efforts of consumer groups concerned with these neurotoxic amino acids that a few people were made aware of the collection sites and the fact that reports of reactions could be sent to the FDA.

The FDA's suppression of information doesn't stop with the toxic potential of MSG. We've found the agency routinely puts the lid on anything that might negatively impact the bottom lines of companies in the food or drug industries. Acid-hydrolyzed proteins, for example, all contain carcinogenic mono and dichloro propanols. Have you seen any warning about ingesting acid-hydrolyzed proteins? Has the FDA done anything to limit the carcinogens in acid-hydrolyzed proteins?

Most, if not all hydrolyzed proteins, are hydrolyzed using acids. Acids break down protein into individual amino acids (including glutamic acid) and unavoidable impurities, including carcinogenic mono and dichloro propanols[158].

Jack verbally advised the FDA in 1993 that acid-hydrolyzed proteins introduced carcinogenic propanols into processed foods. He didn't realize the FDA was already aware of that fact[159]. The December 2, 1996 issue of *Food Chemical News* reported that, "The Food and Drug Administration is working with the hydrolyzed vegetable protein (HVP) industry to address its concerns about the presence of chloropropanols in acid-HVP." The article went on to report that, "Two chloropropanols...are considered genotoxic carcinogens by several international organizations, according to FDA." *Food Chemical News* went on to report that according to Greg Diachenko, director, Division of Product Manufacture and Use in the Center for Food Safety and Applied Nutrition's Office of Premarket Approval, the "FDA has known about the formation of chloropropanols in HVP for some time, but its carcinogenic potential was not known until a few years ago." (That would have been during the mid-1990's).

The Joint Food and Agriculture Organization of the United Nations (FAO/WHO) Expert Committee on Food Additives and Contaminants (JECFA) determined the carcinogenicity of chloropropanols at its 41st meeting, held in February 1993. Another key scientific body, the European Union's Scientific Committee for Food, concluded that levels of 3-MCPD should be reduced to undetectable levels because it had been shown to cause cancer in rats when administered in large doses over long time periods.

To date, I've seen no warnings on labels of foods that contain acid-hydrolyzed proteins, stating that those foods contain carcinogens. I call that suppression of information.

Suppression of information by professionals is not unknown. Suppression of criticism of badly flawed glutamate industry-sponsored research has been extraordinarily effective. Our questions, in the form of letters to the editor refuting articles by Goldschmiedt, Redfern, and Feldman[154] and Daniels and Diachenko[160] have been refused publication by the *American Journal of Clinical Nutrition* and *Food Additives and Contaminants.*

When I sent a critique of the work of Tarasoff and Kelly[73] to *Food and Chemical Toxicology* as a letter to the editor, it was first accepted for publication but subsequently rejected.

In the end, I was informed that their battery of expensive solicitors had assured them that by publishing the letter, the damage to reputation caused by their initial acceptance and then rejection, if any, had been sufficiently allayed[161]. My letter to the editor of *Food and Chemical Toxicology*[73] was published more than a year after publication of the original article.

In case you're looking for the big picture in all this, please note that Dr. Joseph Borzelleca, then editor of *Food and Chemical Toxicology*, was among those who told me the FDA wouldn't be accepting the 1994 Final Draft Report of the "independent" FASEB evaluation of the safety of MSG in food. Borzelleca told me he'd seen the report, and the glutamate industry wasn't pleased with it. Interesting, also, is the fact that Borzelleca was, at that time, on the faculty of the Medical College of

Virginia, while Donald F. Kirby, M.D., was doing double-blind studies for the IGTC at the same institution[162].

The mainstream medical community has been equally complicit in suppressing information that might be of benefit to MSG-sensitive consumers. What physician, dietician or nutritionist will provide patients with the names of the ingredients in which MfG is hidden? We haven't bothered to track much of the glutamate industry influence, but, for example, it's on record as being generous in its support of the American Dietetic Association[163-164].

Allergists are among those most vocal in their endorsements of the safety of MSG and in suppressing information that would say otherwise. They, as a group, refuse to consider that sensitivity to MSG is a reaction to a toxin/poison, not an IgE mediated allergic reaction,[A] and thus they test for MSG sensitivity with inappropriate allergy tests. If not purposefully deceptive and misleading, I consider allergy testing for MSG sensitivity at minimum a form of malpractice.

Endorsement is the other side of the coin. The American Academy of Family Physicians Foundation allowed the IFIC, which does work for the IGTC, to claim "Favorable Review by the American Academy of Family Physicians Foundation" on its 1991 brochure "What you should know about monosodium glutamate."

The bottom line? Interwoven with the assertion that research says monosodium glutamate is "safe," has been the suppression of virtually all commentary or data that would say otherwise. The FDA, the media and the medical community are essentially under glutamate industry control. The "virtually" comes from the fact that the glutamate industry doesn't yet have complete control of the Internet, although search results are easily manipulated to place glutamate industry-friendly pages among the top results.

DISSEMINATION OF DECEPTIVE AND MISLEADING INFORMATION

There's not much difference between endorsement of monosodium glutamate and dissemination of deceptive and/or misleading information. Call it what you want, it's two sides of the same coin with the message on both sides telling consumers it's safe to buy products that contain monosodium glutamate.

The Glutamate Association and IGTC have disseminated masses of misinformation designed to play down reports of adverse or toxic reactions that might catch the eye of physicians or consumers. Their aim is to convince anyone who'll look or listen that monosodium glutamate is safe.

Before 1989 we believed what Ajinomoto wanted us to believe: monosodium glutamate is a functional flavor enhancer with no side effects. We knew Jack reacted to the substance and he wasn't the only one to do so, but we had no idea there were so many others like him. Having read nothing but propaganda provided by the glutamate industry, we believed only a few people reacted to monosodium glutamate, their reactions were mild and transitory, and it would take 5 grams of MSG to cause a reaction. We had no idea how much MSG there was in any product.

By the end of 1989, I'd begun reading everything I could find on the subject of monosodium glutamate. In 1989, we were just starting to consider that not everything the glutamate industry told us was true.

First, we learned that people vary in their sensitivities to monosodium glutamate and the other ingredients that contain the same manufactured free glutamic acid — MfG. Then we actually met a young lady whose reaction was worse than Jack's. She'd been an outstanding high school long distance runner, but in her final year, her migraine headaches became so severe that she'd been hospitalized, and she dropped to last place in competitions. The migraines were only part of the issue, as she became stroke-like, with paralysis on one side of her body. Her face on that side as well as her arm and leg would become contorted. Recovery, although complete, took up to six months with considerable physical therapy. It was ultimately determined that her reactions were caused by exposure to monosodium glutamate.

As we researched Jack's problem, we began to note more and more discrepancies in the information put out by the glutamate industry. Monosodium glutamate, Ajinomoto said, was obviously safe. It had been used in food for over 2,000 years. But we read in the literature of The Glutamate Association and IGTC, both part of Ajinomoto's basic network, that monosodium glutamate was first manufactured in 1908.

The more we read, the more discrepancies we discovered. Slowly, we began to identify the people who were endorsing the safety of monosodium glutamate and disseminating the glutamate industry's deceptive and misleading information. Much of our information came from the writings of The Glutamate Association and IGTC. In 1989 and 1990, they were pleased to brag about monosodium glutamate's endorsements, and cite information disseminated by individuals and organizations speaking in glowing terms about their wonderful product. By the time I published "The toxicity/safety of processed free glutamic acid (MSG): a study in suppression of information,"[8] I had identified various individuals, agencies, organizations, and so-called authoritative bodies that carried their messages of safety.

Some individuals and organizations with alleged interest in food safety reviewed the safety of MSG favorably. Some of their names will be familiar, while others will not: American College of Allergy and Immunology[165-167], Institute of Food Technologists[168], *Mayo Clinic Nutrition Letter*[169], *In Health*[170], Kristin McNutt[171], Patricia Taliaferro[172], *Tufts University Diet and Nutrition Letter*[173], *Modern Maturity*[174], and the *University of California at Berkeley Wellness Letter*[175-176]. Others prepared brochures stating there's no evidence that ingestion of monosodium glutamate or other MSG-containing food additives should cause concern. The American Academy of Allergy and Immunology, the FDA in cooperation with IFIC, and the Scripps Clinic and Research Foundation produced brochures listing a number of food additives that might concern consumers, while omitting any mention of MSG or other MfG-containing ingredients.

Going a step further, the AMA House of Delegates refused to implement Resolution 187, which was adopted at the AMA 1991 Annual Meeting (Policy 150.970, AMA Policy Compendium, 1992 Edition), which called for the AMA to "...encourage all appropriate regulatory agencies, including the Food and Drug Administration, to mandate labeling of all foods containing even small amounts of additive L-glutamic acid so that individuals wanting to avoid this substance may do so."

Depending on the roles they play, researchers might be considered agents of the glutamate industry. In addition, there are those who promote the products of the companies they work for, just as public relations firms do, only these organizations highlight the fact that they're nonprofits while minimizing the fact that they work on behalf of profit-making enterprises. Individuals employed by the IFIC and the International Life Sciences Institute (ILSI) are examples of such glutamate industry agents.

Some of their information is based on distortion of fact. One example would be the statement that the glutamic acid in monosodium glutamate is chemically identical to the glutamic acid found in unadulterated protein. The truth is that monosodium glutamate is a manufactured product that invariably contains D-glutamic acid, pyroglutamic acid and other impurities as well as L-glutamic acid. The glutamic acid found in unadulterated protein is composed only of L-glutamic acid.

Typical is the assertion that "other authoritative bodies" have found MSG to be safe. In general, those other authoritative bodies have read the FDA's summaries concluding that MSG is safe, or have received selected data provided to them by The Glutamate Association and have called that their data. When questioned, Helen Keller International, one of the "authoritative bodies," was not at all pleased to hear that its name was being used in this way. They had never considered that MSG might have toxic potential. Helen Keller International was supplementing monosodium glutamate, a widely used food additive, with vitamin A in Indonesia to counteract xerophthalmia, an eye disease caused by lack of vitamin A. It didn't consider that to be an endorsement of the safety of MSG.

In 1991, faced with the threat of having the toxic potential of monosodium glutamate exposed on *60 Minutes* the IFIC's MSG Committee/MSG Coalition stepped up its activity on behalf of the glutamate industry, producing the "Communication Plan: July-December, 1991" that detailed methods for scuttling the scheduled program, or, failing that, provided for crisis management[177].

According to the *Encyclopedia of Associations*, the IFIC serves as a source of scientific information on food safety and nutrition; disseminates information to the media, the professional health community, and consumers; and seeks to foster the acceptance, growth, and development of MSG[178]. IFIC's paid relationship to the glutamate industry is clearly documented.

The vehicles used to carry the glutamate industry's messages include persons who might be able to influence people in high places (state or federal legislators, for example), press releases, reviews of the safety of monosodium glutamate placed in medical and nutrition journals, and speeches to nutrition and medical groups or any other group that might listen.

Information disseminated about the safety of monosodium glutamate is found in health letters (the *University of California Berkeley Wellness Letter*, for example); targeted journals (such as those focusing on women's issues, children, food, sports, or nutrition); *The FDA Medical Bulletin* (since discontinued); the *FDA Backgrounder*; the *FDA Consumer*; physicians' journals; articles in newspapers and magazines along with TV news features; websites of the IGTC, The Glutamate Association, the International Glutamate Information Service (one of its affiliated organizations), individual agents or cooperating organizations; reviews in nutrition, nursing, and medical journals, and actual paid advertising.

Over the last three decades, the glutamate industry has distributed reams of material designed to convince the public that MSG is safe. In 1989, when consumers raised questions about the safety of free glutamic acid, the FDA commonly referred consumers directly to The Glutamate Association or sent them material prepared by it. In the past, FDA practice included distributing unsolicited copies of an FDA Medical Bulletin that assured physicians MSG is safe, and distributing similar material to food service people. In the January-February 2003 FDA Consumer Magazine, Michelle Meadows, in an article titled "MSG: A Common Flavor Enhancer," spewed out words that give the appearance of having come directly from the IGTC, The Glutamate Association, or the International Glutamate Information Service — trying to convince consumers MSG is safe while really saying nothing.

We've found glutamate propaganda in the most interesting places. If you see an article in a magazine that praises monosodium glutamate or any other MSG-containing product, chances are there will be a paid advertisement from a producer or user of MSG on the same page. There are few medical journals any more that will carry the glutamate industry's badly flawed research. Chances are if you come across a fairly recent article, it will be in a journal that sells advertising.

We've argued that published glutamate industry-sponsored studies are badly flawed. If that's the case, their publication in peer-reviewed journals might be difficult to justify. Consider, however, that if the peers who review the work of glutamate industry representatives are themselves glutamate industry representatives, or very close friends, it's akin to the "fox guarding the henhouse." Consider also that journals such as the *Journal of Allergy and Clinical Immunology* take (or previously took) advertising, and journals such as the *American Journal of Clinical Nutrition* acknowledge the generous support of members of the food and/or drug industries. Both those journals have a history of publishing glutamate industry-sponsored studies.

Glutamate industry representatives and friends also sit on boards of "independent" organizations. I've already mentioned the role Andrew Ebert has played in this area. Glutamate industry researcher and spokesman Ronald Simon has been a member of the Scientific Advisory Board of the Center for Science in the Public Interest (CSPI). Monsanto's Robert Shapiro sits, or sat, on the board of the Tufts University School of Nutrition. Allergy support groups often include industry-friendly allergists on their medical advisory boards. Steve Taylor has served on the Medical Advisory Board of The Food Allergy Network. (When last I inquired, The Food Allergy Network was not providing its members with lists of the hidden sources of MfG. Similarly, "independent organizations" whose medical advisory board members have ties to the glutamate industry have not provided information to their members about MfG-containing ingredients.

Glutamate industry involvement is rarely obvious. That's what makes it so effective. An *In Health* article[170] ran next to an advertisement from McCormick, a member of The Glutamate Association. Had the McCormick ad not been placed so close to the article, the possibility that McCormick might have commissioned the article might have escaped my notice. (Magazines and newspapers often do "advertorials," stories about, or on behalf of, companies that purchase advertising.) Then there's always congenial Andy Ebert, who doesn't mention his ties to monosodium glutamate, Ajinomoto, the IGTC, and now aspartame (a.k.a. AminoSweet, Neotame, NutraSweet, Equal, and E951).

Much of the misinformation circulated by the glutamate industry comes in the form of half-truths. When The Glutamate Association's Richard Cristol wrote to FASEB on April 9, 1993 that researchers had received no funding from The Glutamate Association, he didn't rule out receipt of funding from the IGTC, Ajinomoto, Campbell's or other members of the glutamate industry.

On page five of a brochure titled "Sweet, sour, salty, bitter and umami," put out by the Umami Information Center[179] the statement is made that "... researchers confirmed that glutamate had an L-configuration." While it's true that most glutamate has an L-configuration, it's also true that when glutamate is generated through a manufacturing process or through fermentation, the glutamate produced will contain D-glutamate as well as L-glutamate. Pyroglutamic acid will invariably accompany manufacture, and under certain circumstances, carcinogenic substances will also be generated.

Our favorite example of misinformation is Ajinomoto's use of the concept of umami. What an idea! It's common knowledge among those who work for the glutamate industry that there are receptors in the mouth and on the tongue called glutamate receptors — receptors that are stimulated by free glutamate. So hire a band of researchers to produce studies demonstrating that food containing free glutamate can stimulate those glutamate receptors, and announce to the world that they have discovered a fifth taste, called umami.

Never mind that for years, monosodium glutamate was described as a tasteless white crystalline powder. Never mind that Julia Child, who in her later years was recruited to praise the use of monosodium glutamate, never once mentioned monosodium glutamate in her original cookbook. Never mind that if there was taste associated with monosodium glutamate, people like Jack, who are sensitive to MSG, would be highly motivated to identify it and thereby avoid ingesting MSG — which they claim they can't do.

I have this creeping suspicion that the concept of umami has been marketed in an effort to legitimize the use of monosodium glutamate in food, and draw attention away from the fact that the essential component of monosodium glutamate is a neurotoxic amino acid that kills brain cells, causing obesity and reproductive disorders.

I actually talked once with one of the umami researchers. A friend told me that a biochemist/nutritionist acquaintance on the faculty at UC Davis could help me understand glutamate and monosodium glutamate, but when I called, he explained that he didn't have the expertise I was looking for, and suggested I call Dr. Michael O'Mahoney, professor in the Department of Food Science and Technology, who was doing research for the glutamate industry and, therefore, could certainly help me.

O'Mahoney was warm and friendly, just like Taylor and Cristol had been earlier. He was sorry, he told me, but because he had a contract with Ajinomoto to study the taste of monosodium glutamate, he wasn't able to share information with me.

An academician who refused to share information was an animal I hadn't met before.

A decade ago, what seemed to be the glutamate industry's favorite bit of misinformation was the statement that eating monosodium glutamate isn't any different than eating protein, since both contain L-glutamic acid. We call that fiction because it isn't true, and Ajinomoto knows it isn't true. Ajinomoto knows monosodium glutamate contains impurities that come as a consequence of being manufactured — and protein doesn't. How do we know they know? Because in the files of the FDA we found a 1994 letter from IGTC Chief Executive Officer Yoshi-hisa Sugita, citing a paper related to trace MSG impurities written by governmental scientists in the Central Customs Laboratory, Ministry of Finance of Japan[13] that says so. That shouldn't come as a surprise, because food-grade L-glutamic acid is sometimes defined as 98-99% pure.

Now, when professional journals hesitate to take articles from glutamate industry researchers, the IGTC holds seminars, and/or has researchers present their industry-friendly papers at professional meetings, following which abstracts of those papers are published. Abstracts are then picked up by the glutamate industry's propaganda teams and cited as studies published in peer-reviewed journals, ignoring the fact that only abstracts were published, and the studies being reported on were not peer reviewed. One of the principal forums for such papers has been the *Journal of Allergy and Clinical Immunology*. In addition, there are a few journals that, by policy, don't accept critical letters. *Food Additives and Contaminants* is (or was) one. Regardless of the venue used for publication of glutamate industry reviews or research, this information is made available to the medical community and the media, and assumes great propaganda value.

The potential for glutamate industry influence over the media is obvious. Radio, TV, and newspapers all carry vast amounts of food and drug advertising. Moreover, members of media boards of directors may also be directors of food and/or drug companies.

Whether or not these people and/or organizations act as agents of the glutamate industry or are simply influenced by them is irrelevant. Either way, they publish material that's read by others who respect their opinions, and that material is uncritical of anything said or done by the glutamate industry. Characteristic of those referenced here is their unwillingness to print any addition, correction, or retraction after errors or omissions in published material are pointed out to them.

The scientific community has been given information by the IGTC and The Glutamate Association, and through intermediaries such as IFIC and ILSI, is encouraged to pass it on to the public. Allergists, dieticians and nutritionists appear to have been particularly targeted. Furthermore, the media appear to have been well supplied with glutamate industry materials and to be under tremendous pressure from food and drug advertisers to comment only positively about the value of monosodium glutamate, or not comment at all. IFIC claims that "some three out of four journalists [surveyed] said they use [the IFIC newsletter] *Food Insight* as background for news stories"[180].

DIRTY TRICKS

Maybe they fall into the categories of suppression of information or dissemination of misinformation, but we prefer to call them dirty tricks. We think of suppression of information and dissemination of misinformation as being aimed at the general public, but we take dirty tricks personally.

When we formed the Truth in Labeling Campaign in 1994 our first project was to secure full and clear labeling of MSG. In August 1995, TLC sued the FDA and announced plans for fundraising. In October 1995, the *Washington Post* ran a story about an organization called the Truth in Food Labeling Campaign, formed by Public Voice for Food and Health Policy and the National Consumers League. According to the article, the purpose of the Truth in Food Labeling Campaign was to raise funds to combat the use of mechanically separated poultry (MSP).

How strange is that? Shortly after our group, Truth in Labeling Campaign, announces that we're going to be raising money for labeling MSG, a Truth in Food Labeling Campaign announces that it's going to raise funds to combat MSP.

We thought it was pretty funny, and an innocent coincidence—until the sponsors of the Truth in Food Labeling Campaign refused to reveal the source of the grant money given to them to set up the group, and wouldn't elaborate on projects planned for the future. Would someone have wanted to derail the fundraising efforts of the Truth in Labeling Campaign by forming this oh-so-similar-sounding organization?

To generate publicity for our lawsuit, TLC contracted with Bacons Communications to send out press releases announcing it. However, on the day following the agreed-on distribution date, TLC began to get calls about receipt of incomplete information — received by fax — often only a cover page. As the number of inquiries grew, we confronted Bacons, and found our efforts to generate publicity had been purposely thwarted. It became clear the error wasn't due to a misunderstanding of instructions or equipment breakdown. After a little research, I found food and pharmaceutical companies were among Bacons' regular clients.

In 1994, I attended an IFT Short Course, "Allergies and other Adverse Reactions to Foods, Additives and Ingredients," sponsored by the IFT, The Food Allergy Center, and the University of Nebraska Food Processing Center. Presenters were IGTC spokesperson Daryl Altman, M.D.; Betty P. Rauch, M.B.A., Allerx Inc.; Daniel J. Skrypec, Ph.D., Kraft General Foods; and Sean F. Altekruse, D.V.M., M.P.H., FDA. To my amazement, very little was said about MSG as a trigger of adverse reactions, but what was said was essentially accurate. It was only after the presentation that I discovered that prior to it, Dr. Altman had given members of the press alleged "copies of the presentation" that were replete with misinformation about the safety of MSG. Altman had suggested that reporters didn't need to attend the actual session.

In a letter dated May 28, 1991, the FDA's Dr. Shank cited my letter of December 30, 1990 to FDA Commissioner David Kessler, significantly distorting its text and accusing me of actions I hadn't taken. In September 1995, Dr. Roland Auer wrote to Jack, citing a letter he'd written, significantly distorting its text and accusing him of saying things he hadn't said. Were these distortions set up for some purpose? Were we supposed to get angry and say things we'd later regret? Were we supposed to sue Shank or Auer? Were we supposed to be frightened? Or were they just planning for the future: putting something false into print, and then, if needed later for propaganda purposes, being prepared to quote it as though it were true?

It's already been mentioned that those doing research for the IGTC used aspartic acid (found in aspartame) in their placebos. In anticipation of (or response to) criticism, those in the glutamate industry offered that anyone who'd like to check out the contents of their placebos would be welcome to come to one of their test sites and take a sample placebo from the placebos set aside to allay such concerns.

Generous as it might seem at first reading, this offer actually gave me great cause for concern. Where I come from, a "sample" would be something randomly drawn from a population, and therefore, representative of it. Placebos "set aside" by people who conduct research when components of placebos are in question don't meet anyone's criterion for a randomly drawn sample. Might "set aside placebos" be a dirty trick?

Is a fax machine that falters only when material pertaining to the toxicity of MSG is being transmitted a dirty trick? Given that wire-tapping technology 30 years ago wasn't what it is today, it could have been that our fax line was tapped.

Is it a dirty trick to lie about the nature and severity of MSG reactions? Is it a dirty trick to tell people who might be MSG sensitive to get tested by an allergist when you know the reaction to MSG is a sensitivity reaction, and no traditional allergy test will identify it?

Whatever you call them, we've experienced many. And I suspect we haven't noticed them all.

Most fun was the fax machine. I don't remember what our project was at the time, but along with faxing things to our accountant, we were faxing information of one sort or another to people who were interested in the safety/toxicity of MSG. While the fax seemed to work most of the time, when I'd send a document that had something to do with MSG, or someone would fax a similar document to me, the machine would do a few pages and then stop. I finally got so annoyed that I carried the machine down the hill to a shop where it could be repaired. "Sorry lady," the repairman said, "I can't fix it 'cause it isn't broken."

MARKETING / LOBBYING

According to the American Marketing Association, "Marketing is the activity, set of institutions, and processes for creating, communicating, delivering, and exchanging offerings that have value for customers, clients, partners, and society at large"[181]. When applied by the glutamate industry, it appears that value for customers, clients, partners, and society is defined as activity that leads to the purchase of products that contain MSG.

According to the Free Dictionary, lobbying is "The process of influencing public and government policy at all levels: federal, state, and local"[182].

I think of badly flawed research, suppression of information, dissemination of misinformation, and dirty tricks as parts of the glutamate industry's marketing package. From what we've heard from legislators, it would appear that the message carried to them that MSG is a harmless food additive is built on the components of such a marketing package.

CHAPTER EIGHT NOTES

A. IgE-mediated food allergies are true food allergies involving an abnormal response of the immune system to one or more specific foods. These reactions are associated with the rapid onset of symptoms usually within a few minutes to a few hours after the ingestion of the offending food. Immediate hypersensitivity reactions are mediated by an allergen-specific immunoglobulin E (IgE) antibody. The food allergens involved in IgE mediate reactions are typically naturally occurring proteins in foods. In IgE-mediated food allergies, exposure to the allergen stimulates the production of allergen-specific antibodies by plasma cells in susceptible individuals.

Chapter Nine

The Fail-Safe for Hiding MSG

The genius of Ajinomoto is nowhere better illustrated than in the development of the 3-gram MSG labeling strategy. It would appear that the Glutes had planned from the start to use the 1993 FASEB study (a.k.a. the 1995 FASEB Report) to lay lay the foundation for the big con, pretending to label the MfG in food while leaving most MfG unidentified.

Review of analyses of amounts of MSG in processed foods suggests that half a gram will trigger reactions in most people who are MSG-sensitive. There were a number of independent analyses done some years ago on canned soups which are notorious for causing MSG reactions. Most contained about .6 grams of processed free glutamic acid (MfG) per serving, but none contained as much as 1 gram. Moreover, the label on Accent brand monosodium glutamate states (or stated) that one serving of pure monosodium glutamate is .5 grams of monosodium glutamate.

How much MfG does it take to cause an adverse reaction? No one knows because no one's done a systematic study to provide that information. We do know from published reports of adverse reactions that as little as .5 grams of MSG/MfG can trigger adverse reactions. We also know that some MSG-sensitive people react to the minute amounts of processed free glutamic acid found in binders and fillers of pharmaceuticals — in ingredients with names like maltodextrin and cornstarch. The fact remains that no study to determine the least amount of MSG/MfG that will cause a reaction has ever been done. And even if a study was undertaken, chances are it would be designed to produce meaningless averages and not focus on the individual differences that make up the reactions to MfG.

At the end of the 20th century, the safety of monosodium glutamate was being seriously challenged. The use of aspartame in placebos used in glutamate industry double-blind studies had been exposed, and increasing numbers of consumers were stating that they suffered adverse reactions following ingestion of MfG. Might the glutamate industry be worried? What if someone of stature who had the ear of major media — someone not influenced by the largess of the glutamate industry or friends at Monsanto, or someone not afraid of losing their job or their research funding — spoke out about the toxic effects of MSG, and this information could no longer be effectively suppressed? What if an insider, a whistleblower, came forward?

What if? Not to worry. The glutamate industry's plan to deal with such an eventuality had been set in motion years ago. No longer would industry focus on the claim that essentially no one is sensitive to MSG. Instead, Ajinomoto and friends would agree to labeling some MfG, but not all MfG. Specifically, the MfG in any ingredient or product that contained less than 3 grams of MfG wouldn't be identified on product labels. The claim would be made by the glutamate industry that MSG/MfG was being identified on product labels, while most of the MfG in processed food would go unidentified. By using 3 grams as a basis for labeling, most MfG would remain hidden. Labeling some but not all MfG would cause more confusion than benefit to consumers.

It may have been the work of David Allen, M.D. that first suggested to the glutes that 3.0 grams would be a convenient figure to use as a cutoff point for labeling MSG. Allen had found that 2.5 grams of MSG could trigger asthma, and had published his findings in a peer-reviewed journal[183]. Subsequently, that research (demonstrating that 2.5 grams of MSG/MfG could cause an adverse reaction) would be cited by the glutamate industry as demonstration of the "fact" that 3 grams or more MfG would be **needed** to cause an adverse reaction. The glutamate industry, however, had a problem with using Allen's research results, for Allen had also found that half a gram (.5 grams) of MSG/MfG could trigger asthma — and if that information surfaced, it could kill the 3-gram strategy. So what would Ajinomoto do?

Strategy

1. Cite just that section of Allen's peer-reviewed published study where he reported that 2.5 grams of MSG could trigger asthma. Do not mention the fact that Allen also found that .5 grams of MSG could trigger asthma.

2. Establish a 3-gram figure as the amount — the least amount — of MSG required to cause an MSG reaction as opposed to an amount of MSG that would cause an MSG reaction — obscuring the fact that adverse reactions occur following ingestion of less than 3 grams.

3. Discredit Allen. Once the 3-gram figure was established as the amount that would cause an MSG reaction, the research reported by Allen would be discredited — just in case someone should later refer to the fact that he'd found that .5 grams of MSG/MfG could also cause a reaction.

Implementation: The FDA's 1995 FASEB Report

After the 1994 final report of the "independent study" done for the FDA by FASEB had been found to be inadequate by the IGTC, the FDA had returned what it now called the "draft final report" to FASEB "for clarification." The final report, published in 1995, revealed that "clarification" included stating that it would take 2.5 grams or more of MSG to produce an MSG reaction. When finally published in 1995, the FASEB report on the safety of monosodium glutamate in food read, in part:

> "Despite the fragmented and limited data available, the Expert Panel concluded that there appears to be a subgroup of as yet not fully characterized asthmatic patients that may respond to oral challenges of doses of MSG that exceed 2.5 g per challenge"[93].

FASEB's "independent" report to the FDA had been delivered to the FDA in 1994; found by the Glutes to be unacceptable; and returned by the FDA to FASEB for "clarification." Since our repeated requests for copies of that report were denied, I can only surmise from the information that Borzelleca had shared with me while discussing the

Tarasoff and Kelly study, that the report did not adequately lay the groundwork for the Glutes' planned program for hiding MSG in processed food, and the report had to be modified — which it was.

This FDA move to cooperate with the glutamate industry was not without precedent. In 1978, the glutamate industry had found a study of the Select Committee on GRAS Substances (Evaluation of the Health Aspects of Certain Glutamates as a Food Ingredient) done for the FDA by FASEB[184] to be similarly unacceptable. In response, Ajinomoto and friends had convened a symposium in Milan, Italy, submitted the Milan research reports (primarily glutamate industry sponsored) to the FDA, and had the 1978 FASEB/FDA report rewritten[185].

The FDA's Advanced Notice of Proposed Rulemaking (ANPR)

Following publication of the 1995 FASEB report, the FDA published an Advanced Notice of Proposed Rulemaking (ANPR), citing the 1995 FASEB report as justification for labeling MSG. The extent of FDA/industry cooperation can again be seen in the FDA's substitution of 3 grams or more of MSG needed to cause an adverse reaction for the lesser amount (2.5 grams) published in 1995 by FASEB.

The ANPR summary said in part: "The Food and Drug Administration (FDA) is considering establishing requirements for label information about the free glutamate content of foods. The recent finding of the Federation of American Societies for Experimental Biology (FASEB) that oral ingestion of 3 or more grams (g) of monosodium glutamate (MSG) without food can cause adverse reactions in certain otherwise healthy individuals has prompted the agency to consider what action is necessary to protect consumers from inadvertently ingesting levels of MSG or other forms of free glutamate that could cause an adverse reaction. Thus, the agency seeks public comment..."[186].

The ANPR was not a proposed rule. It was an announcement asking for comments on whether there should be a proposed rule — an announcement made to demonstrate to the judge hearing our lawsuit (Truth in Labeling Campaign, et al., Plaintiffs vs. Donna Shalala, et al., Defendants) that the FDA was evaluating the need to label MSG. While the ANPR docket (96N-0244) remained open, input to the ANPR would not be evaluated, i.e., no action would be considered by the FDA.

With the court's decision to defer to the FDA on the matter of labeling MSG, the FDA dropped much of its pretense of considering labeling. According to a conversation with Dockets Management on January 5, 2009, the ANPR was withdrawn in 2004.

A July 21, 2003 letter from The Glutamate Association to the FDA Dockets Management illustrates the way in which the glutamate people reinforced the deceptive and misleading statements made on their behalf by the FDA. That letter reads in part:

> "The [1996] ANPR was prompted, in significant part, by FDA's interpretation of a 1995 report of the Life Sciences Research Office (LSRO) of the Federation of American Societies for Experimental Biology (FASEB) concerning the safety of [monosodium glutamate] and other glutamate-containing ingredients. FDA interpreted the report to support a conclusion that certain sensitive individuals may experience adverse reactions following the administration of a bolus dose of 3 grams of MSG in a fasting state[187].

Never is it mentioned that a half-gram of MSG has been shown to cause an asthmatic reaction.

Discrediting the Work of Allen
The work of discrediting Allen was left to Simon and Stevenson of Scripps Clinic, La Jolla, California.

Chapter Ten

Your FDA: Guardian of the Glutamate Industry

"A complicating factor in [FDA] evaluation of MSG and glutamates has arisen because a few individuals have very openly questioned the motives and competencies of FDA to provide for the proper scientific review and regulation of this substance....In the past, we have been better able to control the issues we chose to address and the timing."
— Food Chemical News, July 29, 1991, p.25

"It's not that the public is dumb," Shank said. "They need education. We have to find out how to give it to them."
— Food Chemical News, October 28, 1991, p.39

"If the outcome of the review raises substantive questions about the safety of MSG, FDA will require industry to conduct studies to resolve the questions" [Shank] said.
— Food Chemical News, April 20, 1992, p.41

"The FDA's findings were based on the scientific studies provided by the Glutamate Association, according to David Hattan, Ph.D., deputy director for the division of toxicological review and evaluation at the FDA. 'The work has been supported by people with an interest in glutamate: consortiums and manufacturers,' he says."
— Journal of Dental Hygiene, May, 1992, p.158

S ince 1989, much of my time has been spent attempting to have MfG identified wherever and whenever it appears in processed food. That's something I'm still working on.

It is hard to imagine that in 1990 we had thought the FDA looked out for the interests of consumers, guaranteeing them safe food, drink and pharmaceuticals. In the year 2000 we understood that the FDA is nothing more than an extension of industry, promoting the welfare of big business while paying lip service to protecting consumers. When we looked back, neither of us could believe how naïve we were. How for years we gave them the benefit of the doubt. How at every opportunity we gave them the chance to say "we were wrong" or "we were negligent" or "we didn't realize..." But they didn't. It took Jack nearly 20 years to admit that one of the greatest hoaxes played on the American people is the FDA, and the people we elect to public office — Democrats, independents, and Republicans alike — enable them. To the end, Jack had trouble admitting that the evil permeating the FDA permeates a large part of society. He resisted admitting it, even when he knew it was true.

It's the FDA that determines whether monosodium glutamate or any other chemical will be approved for use in food, in whole or with restrictions. It's the FDA that holds the key to changing a product's status. Thus, the FDA also holds the keys to life and death for many Americans, some of whom still believe it's their welfare, not the profits of the food and/or drug industries, that concerns the FDA. The FDA's refusal to require that all MfG in processed food be identified on product labels made it extremely difficult for Jack to live. Actually, the FDA's refusal to require that all MfG in processed food, pharmaceuticals, and dietary supplements be identified on product labels served as Jack's death warrant.

My first contact with the FDA came in 1989, when Jack, with other MSG-sensitive people, testified before a committee taking input relevant to the proposed National Education and Labeling Act (NLEA). It was there that we met Barbara Mullarkey, who'd introduce us to the Nutrition for Optimal Health Association (NOHA) and the FDA's Adverse Reactions Monitoring System (ARMS).

At one time, ARMS was managed by Rear Admiral Linda Tollefson. In the 1990s, her job included collecting unsolicited reports of adverse reactions to MSG and aspartame. The 1997 reports, which I believe were ARMS' last MSG and aspartame reports, indicated there had been 7,259 reports of reactions to aspartame[188] and 717 reports of adverse reactions to MSG[157]. Tollefson's job didn't include soliciting reports of adverse reactions to MSG or aspartame[189].

Symptoms attributed to MSG in complaints submitted to FDA

REPORTED SYMPTOMS	NO. OF REPORTS	% OF REPORTS	% OF COMPLAINTS
Headache	315	43.9%	17.9%
Vomiting and Nausea	136	19.0%	7.7%
Diarrhea	104	14.5%	5.9%
Abdominal Pain and Cramps	95	13.2%	5.4%
Change in Mood Quality or Level	93	13.0%	5.3%
Change in Heart Rate	90	12.6%	5.1%
Dizziness or Problems with Balance	63	8.8%	3.6%
Difficulty Breathing	59	8.2%	3.4%
Fatigue, Weakness	54	7.5%	3.1%
Localized Pain or Tenderness	46	6.4%	2.6%
Sleep Problems	44	6.1%	2.5%
Change in Sensation (Numbness, Tingling)	42	5.9%	2.4%
Change in Body Temperature	41	5.7%	2.3%
Change in Vision	40	5.6%	2.3%
Change in Activity Level	35	4.9%	2.0%
Chest Pain	34	4.7%	1.9%
Local Swelling	32	4.5%	1.8%
Difficulty Swallowing	25	3.5%	1.4%
Joint and Bone Pain	23	3.2%	1.3%
Changes in Skin and Nail Colorations	21	2.9%	1.2%
Blood Pressure Changes	21	2.9%	1.2%
Other Neurological	21	2.9%	1.2%
Other symptoms (reported by less than 20 complainants)	331	--	18.80%

Symptoms attributed to aspartame in complaints submitted to FDA

REPORTED SYMPTOMS	NO. OF REPORTS	% OF REPORTS	% OF COMPLAINTS
Headache	1900	28.7%	18.9%
Dizziness / Poor Equilibrium	749	11.3%	7.5%
Change in Mood	679	10.3%	6.8%
Vomiting or Nausea	669	10.1%	6.7%
Abdominal Pain and Cramps	466	7.0%	4.6%
Change in Vision	374	5.7%	3.7%
Diarrhea	345	5.2%	3.4%
Seizures and Convulsions	298	4.5%	3.0%
Memory Loss	273	4.1%	2.7%
Fatigue, Weakness	251	3.8%	2.5%
Other Neurological	233	3.5%	2.3%
Rash	227	3.4%	2.3%
Sleep Problems	205	3.1%	2.0%
Hives	194	2.9%	1.9%
Change in Heart Rate	193	2.9%	1.9%
Change in Sensation (Numbness, Tingling)	178	2.7%	1.8%
Itching	177	2.7%	1.8%
Grand Mal	174	2.6%	1.7%
Local Swelling	119	1.8%	1.2%
Difficulty Breathing	117	1.8%	1.2%
Change in Activity Level	115	1.7%	1.1%
Oral Sensory Changes	112	1.7%	1.1%
Change in Menstrual Pattern	107	1.6%	1.1%
Other Skin	103	1.6%	1.0%
Localized Pain and Tenderness	101	1.5%	1.0%
Symptoms reported by less than 100 complainants	1678	.25%	16.7

Some consumers described more than one symptom attributed to aspartame.

Since reading the studies done by Olney and others, I had understood that the manufactured free glutamic acid (MfG) found in monosodium glutamate and the aspartic acid found in the sugar substitute aspartame were neurotoxic amino acids that killed brain cells in the hypothalamus when fed to the very young. In reading the lists of adverse reactions compiled by ARMS[157,188] I came to realize that the adverse reactions listed for monosodium glutamate were not only essentially the same as those listed for aspartame, but occurred with the same relative frequency.

Migraine headache was the most frequently reported reaction for both monosodium glutamate and aspartame.

At one point Jack wrote to then FDA commissioner Dr. David Kessler pointing out that his reactions to MSG were life threatening. Sometime later, Jack received a call from an FDA employee named Meryl, indicating that she'd been assigned to look into his reported life-threatening sensitivity to MSG. Meryl wished to schedule a visit.

At the time, Jack was still traveling for business, and suggested setting an appointment for a time in the future. That seemed to upset the FDA investigator, for she became rude, commenting that she didn't know why she was being asked to do such a review, because it was clear MSG was safe.

Jack must have challenged Meryl's rudeness, because she apologized. She was sorry for being short with him. Her daughter had recently developed some strange undiagnosed condition, and from time to time was rushed to the emergency room from school. She was calling from the hospital.

Jack being Jack, he thought Meryl might feel better if they just chatted a few minutes. Besides, he was always interested in ascertaining if an undiagnosed illness could be related to ingestion of MSG. It wasn't long before Jack determined that Meryl's daughter's problem was, indeed, likely induced by MSG.

Was there any pattern to these occurrences? "Yes," she said, "there was a pattern." On many evenings her daughter went out with the girls, and the previous evening she'd gone out for pizza, as she often did the night preceding an "attack."

What kind of pizza? "Always sausage pizza." Sausage pizza? Sausage pizza, at least in Chicago, typically contained monosodium glutamate or ingredients like autolyzed yeast and natural flavoring that contain hidden MfG. Jack suggested Meryl's daughter might have the same problem he had, and offered to mail information, including a list of the ingredients in which MfG could be hidden, and the types of food in which MfG would most commonly be found.

Eventually Meryl came to Jack's office for his scheduled interview, and quite naturally, Jack asked how her daughter was doing.

"Fine and thank you for asking," came the response. Then, without warning, she blurted out, "Mr. Samuels, you were right. My daughter is

MSG sensitive. As long as she stays away from MSG, she doesn't have these reactions. This report, your medical report, has to be very strong because something has to be done about this," and Meryl proceeded to take Jack's comments.

Jack heard from Meryl again several weeks later. She told Jack she'd visited his family physician, who was acutely aware of his MSG problem. She told Jack his physician had told her he'd been monitoring Jack's stress test when Jack had collapsed. For breakfast, Jack had eaten cereal that contained a very small amount of MSG. Meryl also told Jack that she'd completed her report, and because of the importance of the issue, she wanted Jack to review it to make sure she hadn't missed or misstated anything.

Jack returned his edited report to Meryl when they next met. "This is exactly how it will go in," Meryl said. "This has to be a very strong report."

Sometime later, Jack dropped in to the FDA to visit Dr. Linda Tollefson. Jack had wanted to talk to her, but had never been able to reach her. He wanted to confront her with the fact that every time we wrote to her on an issue related to MSG, her responses would be unrelated to our letters. Finding it impossible to set up a meeting, he simply decided to drop by.

Jack had never gone to the FDA uninvited, and had failed to consider that an invitation might be required. He found, however, that he could easily secure a pass to the second-floor library, take an elevator to the second floor, and continue on to the basement where he knew he could find Tollefson. Since Tollefson had no secretary, he just walked into her office and introduced himself.

"I'd just like to talk with you and say a few things," was what Jack said to a shocked Linda Tollefson, who apparently knew who Jack was before he told her.

"Dr. Tollefson, you keep saying that no one reacts to MSG. Are you prepared to tell me that the report done by one of your employees indicated that I'm not MSG sensitive?"

"Absolutely," she replied, "and in fact your doctor doesn't think you're MSG sensitive, either."

"That's a lie," Jack responded, at which time Tollefson ran from the room, slamming the door. If her statement was accurate, Meryl's report had been changed between the time Jack had seen it and the time it had gotten to Tollefson's desk — just like the minutes of Jack's 1989 meeting with the FDA in Washington had been changed.

Tollefson could have worked directly, instead of indirectly, for industry. Friends who believed aspartame should be pulled from the market advised us that they'd also attempted to talk with Tollefson, who always greeted them with a can of diet soda in hand. Moreover, while she seemed to listen, she never did more than listen to their words and, in turn, explain that aspartame was harmless.

I wrote to FDA Commissioner Kessler at the time, asking that Tollefson be released from her position since she was serving the industry, not consumers. In reply, I was told Tollefson was a faithful servant of the FDA (which I read as "the FDA and the glutamate industry"), and our accusations were unfounded.

Eventually, Tollefson was moved from ARMS and promoted to another position within the agency. Rear Admiral Tollefson became director of the FDA Regional Office in Europe stationed at the U.S. Mission to the European Union in Brussels, where she was responsible for all FDA operations in Europe. I often wonder what messages she carried about the safety of aspartame (AminoSweet/Neotame) and MSG.

Our friend Barbara Mullarkey had studied the reports prepared by Tollefson, and noted a relatively large number of reactions reported in a category titled "other." Barbara filed a Freedom of Information (FOI) request for detail of the category "other," and discovered that four deaths attributed to ingestion of aspartame had been sequestered under "other." "The Ultimate Other," Barbara called it in an article she wrote.

Toward the end of the 1990s, collection of reports on adverse events triggered by aspartame was discontinued. Barbara told us an FDA employee told her it really wasn't necessary to bother the FDA with additional reports of aspartame sensitivity because the FDA knew aspartame was safe. Collection of reports on MSG reactions was similarly discontinued.

A friend and NOHA member who lived near us had an experience similar to the experience Jack had. Her daughter had such severe asthma attacks that she'd been hospitalized a number of times, and, in fact, had almost died on several occasions. The mother had determined that the asthma attacks always followed exposure to MSG, and she was deathly afraid of letting the child eat outside of their home. After one attack, she'd been so upset that she wrote a nasty letter to FDA Commissioner Kessler, decrying the fact that the FDA's inaction was placing her daughter at risk. After sending the letter, she called Jack, and in a trembling voice, said, "I think I did a terrible thing. I wrote this nasty letter while I was really upset and I'm afraid now that I'm going to get in trouble for what I said."

It was not long after that letter was written that an FDA investigator visited the family and interviewed the child's physician. As Jack recalled, the investigator spent three days doing his review, after which our friend called Jack and said, "You'll be so pleased. This man was very polite and he did in fact visit my physician, and when he finished his review, he stopped by the house to again thank me for my cooperation. He told me I'd be very pleased, because he found that without question my daughter was MSG sensitive and it was a serious matter and the report would go in accordingly." Jack told our friend that based on past experience, he found it hard to believe that there would be a report confirming her daughter's asthma was caused by MSG. Jack suggested she wait a month or two and make a FOI request for a copy of the report.

Several months had gone by when Jack received a call from an extremely angry woman. She'd done what Jack suggested, and had received the report, which stated her daughter wasn't reacting to MSG. The report said there was a lot of dust in the house and the asthma was likely the result of poor housekeeping.

As our understanding of the FDA grew, we became aware that in addition to ARMS, the FDA had a Food Advisory Committee in which we should be interested. Jack was still working when notice came that the FDA was putting together this committee and two of its positions would be occupied by non-industry individuals who weren't scientists.

Someone, whose name escapes me, entered Jack's name for one of the consumer positions. He filled out an application after getting some information from Jack, who was happy to cooperate.

Quite a while later, Jack received a call from a man named Nate who introduced himself as an FDA employee. Nate said he'd been assigned to determine if Jack's qualifications fit the requirements for this advisory committee position, but he was in Milwaukee and very busy, so he really didn't want to drive to Chicago to waste his time interviewing Jack. Nate wanted Jack to know that he likely didn't meet the requirements for the position and Nate wasn't going to proceed with his application.

When it was Jack's turn to speak, he asked what was required of a candidate, and Nate told Jack they needed someone who could understand scientific terms. In response, Jack suggested that since he was a science major at Northwestern University and held an advanced degree in hospital administration, including work in public health and science, his understanding of scientific terms should be more than satisfactory.

"But we need someone who can communicate well with physicians and other people in science," Nate said, to which Jack responded that as an administrator who'd successfully operated hospitals, he wouldn't have been successful if he hadn't been able to communicate with physicians.

"Well, the person has to be able to read reports regarding scientific matters and understand them," Nate said, to which Jack simply replied, "I guess you don't understand what hospital administrators do and the training they have."

"OK," said Nate, "I'll put in the report of this interview."

Jack didn't hear from the FDA about the Food Advisory Committee, but did eventually see it announced that appointments to the FDA Food Advisory Committee had been made. The two positions had been filled by IGTC president Ebert, and an Evanston, Illinois woman nutritionist who traveled the country as a representative of the IGTC to advise people that MSG is safe. Jack did two things. First, he sent in a freedom of information act request for the curriculum vitae of all the people who'd applied for the committee. Interestingly enough, there was no paperwork for Jack, and when he questioned the absence of his application, he was told that since paperwork for Jack Samuels didn't exist, he must not have applied.

Second, he wrote a letter to FDA Commissioner Kessler protesting both the destruction of his application and the appointment of the chairman of the IGTC, a trade organization representing the glutamate industry, to a position ostensibly set aside for a consumer advocate. Jack received no reply.

FDA Commissioner Kessler had an interesting management style. He never responded to letters from consumers. When Jack wrote to him directly, he had someone else reply. Lawrence Lin, Ph.D. was evidently assigned to respond to Jack's phone calls and mail, placate him, and keep him off of everyone else's back.

Jack's first response from Lin demonstrated Lin's ignorance of MSG. Jack wrote Kessler accordingly, suggesting that if he was going to assign someone to correspond with him, it would be appreciated if that someone knew what he was talking about.

In the early 1990s Jack had a great deal to say to Kessler, and Lin responded to all of it. Jack would tell you that over time they became friends, because Lin certainly did appear to care about Jack's welfare.

I'll tell you that Lin was simply doing his job as directed: dealing with Jack so no one else had to. I think of Lin like so many others: doing what he was told, staying out of trouble at the FDA, and thereby keeping his job.

The FDA's David Hattan, Ph.D. played a different role. Hattan wasn't charged with placating us. His role was much more important; it appears that he was to represent the interests of the glutamate industry without necessarily appearing to do so. I think Jack was being generous when he said he considered Hattan to be intellectually dishonest.

Hattan knew full well that MSG was neurotoxic and caused adverse reactions. In August 1990, he told a toxicology forum in Aspen, Colorado that glutamic acid was implicated in a number of disease conditions. According to Hattan, "developing data on exogenous and endogenous excitogens or excitotoxins has been the primary spur to the FDA's review of monosodium glutamate."

Hattan had noted the similarity of domoic acid (which as a contaminant in Canadian mussels led to 12 people having permanent losses of memory and three deaths), and glutamate, and was quoted as saying, "It has been theorized that if chronic exposure to environmental excitotoxins can cause neuronal degeneration that is gradually manifested across months or years, it may be possible for natural or endogenous excitatory neurotransmitters like glutamic acid to mediate neuronal degeneration in the central nervous system through some type of slow, possibly accumulative, process."

In May 1992, the *Journal of Dental Hygiene* cited Hattan saying, "The FDA's findings were based on the scientific studies provided by The

Glutamate Association. The work has been supported by people with an interest in glutamate: consortiums and manufacturers."

In 1993, Hattan, then FDA Deputy Director for the Division of Toxicological Review and Evaluation, was FDA liaison to the FASEB study on the safety of monosodium glutamate in food, a position from which he defended the assertion that MSG is safe for human consumption. The discrepancy between Hattan's earlier statements (1990 and 1992) and the role he played during the FASEB study were reminiscent of researchers Auer and Kenney, who first found that monosodium glutamate might have toxic potential, and subsequently proclaimed that it was safe.

Once Hattan assumed the role of FDA/FASEB liaison, any questions he might have had about the toxic potential of MSG disappeared, or at least disappeared from sight. At the end of 1992, it appeared that Hattan was an officer in the army assigned to keep MSG hidden in food, and keep the glutamate industry's cash cow protected. We thought it very likely that he was taking orders from someone who ranked higher than he did in the FDA/industry army.

Over the years, Jack met personally with three FDA commissioners or acting commissioners and corresponded with acting Commissioner Bill Benson who was, in Jack's opinion, the most responsive. Jack also got to know the head of the Center for Food Safety and Applied Nutrition. Every time they met, they'd have cordial discussions. At one time, Jack was invited to Dr. Shank's office, and he brought along a bottle of Bragg's Aminos. For years, this product had prominently displayed the words "No MSG" on the label, when in fact it was nothing more than hydrolyzed soy protein, which would invariably contain manufactured free glutamic acid (MfG). Shank looked at the label and laughed. "Jack, you're wasting your time. You know we're not going to do anything about this."

Commissioners, acting commissioners and department heads all were cordial — and all were beholden to the glutamate industry.

As previously noted, while in Washington to give testimony to the FASEB Expert Panel evaluating the safety of MSG, we'd discovered that copies of most everything going in or out of the FDA, other than classified material, was kept at its Dockets Management Office. We visited Dockets each time we were in Washington and took away copies of interesting papers. We also ordered copies of papers from home, which would be sent to us. As we read and reread the material we gathered, not even Jack could deny the close working relationship that had been forged between the glutamate industry and the FDA. At the end of the day we had observed that:

The glutamate industry, led by Ajinomoto, understood that if all MfG in all processed food was labeled, consumers would be able to determine whether or not an MfG-containing ingredient or product caused them to have irritable bowel syndrome, skin rash, migraine headache, seizures or any other adverse reaction.

Why would that be important? Because if consumers were able to identify the MfG in the things they used and the food they consumed, the fact that asthma, dizziness, and/or depression, for example, always followed MfG use might become obvious. The glutamate industry wouldn't like that at all. It might make it difficult to sell consumers — or maybe even the medical community — on the idea that MfG is harmless.

The FDA cooperated with the glutamate industry at every turn. Its cooperation can be traced back to September 1969, when FDA Commissioner Herbert L. Ley Jr. testified before the Senate Select Committee on Nutrition and Health, presenting evidence from four studies that, he alleged, demonstrated MSG was safe. It was later disclosed that two of those studies were incomplete, and two didn't even exist.

There were no meaningful regulations for identifying MfG or the amount of MfG in any product. The FDA's refusal to identify MfG through labeling is central to the success of the glutamate industry. Where MSG or MfG is concerned, that's really what the FDA is all about.

We'd seen that the FDA allowed "monosodium glutamate" to be given as an illustration of a common safe food:

"It is impracticable to list all substances that are generally recognized as safe for their intended use. However, by way of illustration, the Commissioner regards such common food ingredients as salt, pepper, sugar, vinegar, baking powder, and monosodium glutamate as safe for their intended use." (CFR 21 582.1)

The FDA had acknowledged that to advertise products as "No MSG," "No Added MSG," or "No MSG Added" when they contain ingredients that are sources of free glutamic acid such as hydrolyzed protein, was in direct violation of Section 403(a)(1) of the Federal Food, Drug, and Cosmetic Act. Yet, the FDA allowed the words "No added MSG" and "No MSG added" to be used, illegally, on labels of foods that contain MfG.

The FDA ignored evidence of monosodium glutamate toxicity — or if not ignored completely, evidence of possible MfG toxicity would be submitted to representatives of the glutamate industry for evaluation, whereupon the safety of MSG/MfG would be confirmed.

FDA-sponsored investigations into the safety of monosodium glutamate were rigged from the get-go.

When the glutamate industry wasn't satisfied with the outcome of an FDA investigation, the final report of that investigation would be rewritten.

The FDA cooperated with Ajinomoto in designing studies from which the industry would claim to have demonstrated that MSG was a safe food additive. We found evidence to that effect in the files of the FDA.

The FDA ignored the fact that studies presented to it by the IGTC as evidence that MSG was a harmless food additive used MSG-containing ingredients other than monosodium glutamate as well as neurotoxic aspartic acid (found in aspartame) in their placebos.

The FDA Adverse Reactions Monitoring System (ARMS) was nothing more than window dressing. Among other things, it never solicited information. The FDA disbanded the ARMS when the need to pretend it was interested in the toxic potential of MSG and aspartame diminished.

Minutes of FDA meetings with consumers were changed when it served the purposes of the glutamate industry.

Medical evaluations of MSG-sensitive people were altered by the FDA.

The FDA had chosen two friends of the glutamate industry, IGTC Chairman Ebert and another IGTC operative, to serve as consumer advocates on its Food Advisory Committee.

The FDA suppressed information pertaining to the toxic potential of MSG.

In 1992, the FASEB study on the safety of amino acids in dietary supplements had warned about the use of MfG in supplements. That information was never shared with the public.

As early as 1990, the FDA became aware that MSG produced through acid hydrolysis of proteins contains carcinogenic mono and dichloro propanols. We knew if enzymes were used to produce hydrolyzed proteins, this wouldn't be the case, but since using enzymes is more costly than using acid, it's likely most of the hydrolyzed protein products found in processed foods contribute to the development of cancer.

That information was never shared with the public. Since 1990, the FDA has been thinking about sharing it.

The FDA published and distributed material that they claimed attested to the safety of monosodium glutamate, but did not do so. We saw some of that material in the *FDA Medical Bulletin* and more in the *FDA Backgrounder*.

The FDA reinforced the misinformation put out by the glutamate industry, distortions of fact like, "The glutamic acid in monosodium glutamate is identical to the glutamic acid in whole protein."

The FDA refused to produce documents requested under discovery when sued over its failure to require identification of MSG/MfG through labeling.

When Dockets copied material we'd requested, they made extra copies for Dr. Lin.

The FDA approved the use of glutamate-blocking pharmaceuticals while encouraging industry to pour processed free glutamate into processed food.

The FDA refused to provide consumers with lists of ingredients that contain MfG.

The FDA allowed the term "natural" to be used in reference to excitatory amino acids.

The FDA allowed the glutamate industry to create and use sources of MfG that contain carcinogenic mono and dichloro propanols and heterocyclic amines.

The FDA told people that the free glutamic acid in processed food is identical to the free glutamic acid found in unprocessed food and in higher organisms, without reference to the fact that the free glutamic acid in processed food is invariably accompanied by impurities.

We knew the FDA cooperated with Ajinomoto in designing studies from which the industry would claim to have demonstrated that MSG was a safe food additive. We found evidence to that effect in the files of the FDA, that include:

- A July 13, 1990 letter from IGTC chairman Ebert to Walter Glinsmann, M.D., Associate Director of Clinical Nutrition, Division of Nutrition, FDA reads, in part "...attached are three [double-blind] protocols for your use...IGTC would be interested in your views, especially on the proposed work by Drs. Kirby and Kjos"190.

- A January 2, 1991 letter from IGTC chairman Ebert to Fred R. Shank, Ph.D., Director, Center for Food Safety and Applied Nutrition, FDA, requested a scientific review session on MSG with FDA scientists. IGTC chairman Ebert elaborated on what the IGTC wanted covered at the meeting, and offered the names of FDA personnel who should attend: "In the past, IGTC has requested meetings with FDA staff for purposes of informal reviews of MSG research. Scientists who have carried out studies on MSG, usually in university laboratories or clinics, have presented their data to agency scientists for review and discussion....If Dr. Donald Kirby, who is currently carrying out research on MSG at the Medical College of Virginia, has sufficient clinical data by the time of an FDA meeting we would propose inviting him also."

  After elaborating on what the IGTC wanted covered at the meeting, the chairman continued: "As FASEB plans a one-day Hearing on Free Amino Acids on February 4, 1991, it seems advisable to complete an FDA meeting prior to that date....FDA scientists who have participated in MSG research discussion in the past included among others: Drs. Shank, Hattan and Scheuplein. Others who would be key attendants include Drs. Rulls, Lin and Bailey...Members of the IGTC/TGA Executive Committee also would plan to join the meeting"191.

- A December 9, 1991 FDA Memorandum of Conference notes that "The IGTC requested the meeting to discuss a protocol that they are currently developing for a proposed food allergy study involving MSG. We informed the visitors that we will provide our comments only after they have submitted a written protocol to us with some detailed description of the proposed study."

- A September 4, 1992 FDA Memorandum of Conference that reads: "Dr. Kimura gave me a copy of the [IGTC] request (dated 8/20/92) for a meeting with the Commissioner and a copy of the Bob MacLeod's brief response (dated 9/3/92) to the IGTC. We both agreed that once a description of their research plan (or protocols) is given to us, a meeting will be scheduled for their scientists to discuss with our review staff regarding their research plan aimed to resolve scientific issues surrounding adverse reactions allegedly caused by monosodium glutamate consumed in food."

- Reference to an October 23, 1992 conference hosted by the FDA at its Center for Food Safety and Applied Nutrition. Present were Raif S. Geha (Harvard Medical School), Andrew Saxon (UCLA Medical School), Roy Patterson (Northwestern University Medical School), Ebert, (Chairman IGTC), Yoshi-hisa Sugita (IGTC), Takeshi Kimura (IGTC); and Hattan, Tollefson, Glinsmann, Bailey, and Lin of the FDA. Protocols for the Geha, Saxon, Patterson study called for use of aspartame in placebos, as had all other double-blind studies receiving FDA approval[192].

It was not until the FDA refused to address the January 4, 2021 Citizen Petitions requesting the MSG and MfG be removed from the FDA's GRAS list, and refused to respond to a Freedom of Information request for copies of data used by the FDA for determining to give GRAS status to free glutamic acid used in food and to monosodium glutamate and other ingredients that contain free glutamic acid, that we recognized that the FDA used one of the glutamate-industry's tried and true strategies for hiding the truth about toxic MfG: refusal to answer questions and refusal to address a subject that might suggest that MSG and MfG are toxic.

In 2009 we thought that with the Obama administration, care might be taken to turn the FDA back to its original charge of guaranteeing the safety of both food and drugs. With the appointment of Michael R. Taylor, former partner in the law firm of King & Spalding, and former vice president for public policy of Monsanto Company, to Obama's transition team and from there to the post of FDA Deputy Commissioner for Foods, all hope for a return to concern for consumers disappeared.

Taylor is a cousin of Tipper Gore, the former wife of Al Gore, vice president under President Bill Clinton. The work experience he brings to his most recent job at the FDA comes from years of dedicated service to Monsanto.

Taylor is also the man from President Clinton's FDA who oversaw FDA approval of rBGH (recombinant bovine growth hormone), and thereby subjected citizens of this country, and many others, to increased risk of breast, prostate, and colon cancer. Genetically engineered, rBGH is a potent variant of the natural growth hormone produced by cows. Its use forces cows to increase their milk production by about 10 percent, makes cows sick, and facilitates the production of milk that's chemically and nutritionally different than natural milk.

Taylor has additional glutamate industry credits. He was instrumental in securing FDA approval of aspartame.

Those who viewed the November 3, 1991 *60 Minutes* segment on MSG may remember Taylor's performance in which he represented the interests of the FDA and Ajinomoto (a close friend of Monsanto) as he responded to Mike Wallace's questions. All Taylor would say was that the FDA was looking into labeling. The FDA doesn't even pretend to do that anymore.

On January 14, 2010, Lyndsey Layton wrote an excellent article on Michael Taylor for the *Washington Post* covering every aspect of his professional career, including the following:

> "Taylor is a familiar figure at the FDA. He began his career
> as a staff attorney at the agency in 1976. Then he worked
> for a decade at King & Spalding, which represented

Monsanto Corp., the agribusiness giant that developed genetically engineered corn, soybeans and bovine growth hormone.

He returned to the FDA in 1991 as deputy commissioner for policy and pushed through requirements that producers of seafood and juices adopt measures to prevent bacterial contamination. During the same period, the FDA approved Monsanto's bovine growth hormone, and Taylor was partly responsible for a controversial policy that said milk from BGH-treated cows did not have to be labeled as such.

In 1994, Taylor went to the U.S. Agriculture Department to run its food-safety program. He required meat and poultry producers to take measures to prevent bacterial contamination, despite strong opposition from those industries. Observers expected Taylor to impose those same kinds of preventive controls on all the foods regulated by the FDA.

After the USDA, Taylor went to work for Monsanto as a vice president for public policy. He moved on to a think tank and then a teaching stint at George Washington University.

'He is the quintessential revolving door,' said Marion Nestle, a professor of nutrition, food studies and public health at New York University. Taylor's support for BGH and Monsanto's other genetically modified products at the FDA was 'questionable,' she said. 'On the other hand, when he went to USDA, what he did there was absolutely heroic. He's been very strong on food safety.'"

You might notice, as I have, that the measures Taylor took at the USDA to promote food safety didn't negatively impact Monsanto. Similarly, nothing he was advertised as scheduled to act on as FDA

Deputy Commissioner for Foods would impact Monsanto negatively. I'd also submit that in cases other than those where the role of big business is undeniable, this sort of regulation will be aimed at small, generally independent companies, but protecting the American population from toxic additives intentionally added to processed food won't even be considered. Enforcing regulations prohibiting deceptive and misleading labeling, such as claims that there's no MSG or MfG added to products that contain it, is something that will never happen while the foxes like Michael Taylor are in charge of guarding the henhouse.

I'll never understand how a man who promotes the use of toxic chemicals in processed food can be characterized as devoted to food safety. But I do understand how he got to the FDA in the first place, and what power enabled him to remain there as long as he did. In truth, he never really left Monsanto.

To quote a little phrase I heard on public radio that suits the FDA to a T, "A lap dog, not a watch dog." And neither the president nor the Congress ever walks that dog.

Chapter Eleven

Moving Into a New Decade

I t was all over. We'd learned that the FDA worked hand in glove with the glutamate industry, led by Ajinomoto. We'd come to the FDA with reproducible data attesting to the toxicity of MSG, and been ignored.

We had learned that Ajinomoto and friends were rich and powerful, powerful enough to control the U.S. Congress, any state legislature that might think to challenge them, and for all intents and purposes, control the media. We understood their propaganda campaigns and knew exactly how they rigged the studies they presented to the FDA and "other authoritative bodies" as evidence that their product, monosodium glutamate, was safe. We'd sued the FDA over the issue of labeling, and seen our case dismissed by Magistrate Mummert. In 1989, Jack delighted in the thought that life would soon be better, that he could avoid ingesting the substance that caused him so much suffering. But 10 years later, he had all he could do just to stay alive. A feeling of well-being — good health — was out of the question. He knew there were others like him, others who knew less than he did about avoiding MfG hidden in processed food, but it was small consolation that he was not the only one.

On March 24, 1998, we were at Stanford for Jack's prostate cancer checkup. Everything looked good. He thought it would.

NIH CONFERENCE
From May 3-5, 1998, we attended the NIH-sponsored glutamic acid conference titled, "The Glutamate Cascade; Common Pathways of Central Nervous System Disease States," then spent an additional two days in Washington. I had submitted a presentation to the conference poster session, one that wasn't accepted. That came as no surprise, since

it was already clear there were researchers at the NIH with glutamate industry interests.

We saw a poster presentation, "The Role of Monosodium L-Glutamate (MSG) in Asthma: Does it Exist?" by Donald D. Stevenson funded by the IGTC — done at the time Ronald Simon was swearing that he and Stevenson weren't doing research for the glutamate industry. (That was just another little lie. One not nearly as significant as most of the others.)

STILL TRAVELING

In June 1998, we took a seven-day trip to Atlanta, home of the Kellen Company, the IGTC and anti-aspartame activist Betty Martini.

That year we also went to the Czech Republic, a country Jack had always wanted to visit, since many of his ancestors came from that part of the world. Jack proposed to lay out an itinerary and rent a car as we so often did when we traveled, but I insisted that since neither of us read nor spoke the language, and wouldn't be able to order food in restaurants, we weren't going unless we went with either a tour or a private guide and driver. We decided on the latter; Mirek was our guide, driver, and wonderful traveling companion.

We stayed in private apartments, vacant summer homes, motels and hotels. Mirek found a relative of Jack's who'd survived the Holocaust because his Jewish grandfather, who died just before the Nazis took over the area in which he lived, had married a Catholic girl and converted. We had a long afternoon visit.

Best of all, except for the one reaction Jack had to canned whipped cream, he didn't have an eating problem as long as we were with Mirek.

We closed out 1998 with a trip to Southeast Asia arranged by Archaeological Tours. We traveled from Bangkok through Laos, Cambodia, Burma, and back to Thailand. Jack had to work with our guide the first day to get him to understand Jack's food sensitivity, but from that day forward, there was never a problem. But then, there never is a problem when fresh food is available.

It was particularly easy to avoid MSG in Myanmar because the woman in charge of tourism for the government was severely affected by MSG, and she'd advised restaurants not to use it. We also heard that a physician with political connections had appeared on television, advising citizens to avoid using MSG because it could affect their health. Relative to what was to be found in the United States, Myanmar didn't offer ultra-processed food.

It was about this time that I began working on a web page for the Truth in Labeling Campaign.

UNDER THE RADAR

There were other things happening in 1998 under the radar. On February 8, a friend sent me an e-mail, telling me that the journal *Accountability in Research* had sent out a request for contributions regarding scientific fraud and related issues. My friend thought it would be nice to get some of the stuff the MSG and aspartame industries pass off as research discussed openly in a scholarly journal, and he gave me the e-mail address of the contact somewhere on the other side of the world.

My 51-page article, "The Toxicity/Safety of Processed Free Glutamic Acid (MSG): A Study in Suppression of Information" was published in *Accountability in Research* in July 1999. It had been almost a year and a half in the writing, with my editor insisting that every detail be substantiated. Not once during that time had I mentioned the article on either the phone or the fax; and it is to those restrictions that I attribute the fact that there was no pressure on the publisher to prevent it from being published. But neither was there the open discussion hoped for once the article was published. The glutes and their media simply ignored it.

AUXIGRO

In 1998, there were also things happening that would materially affect us, about which we knew nothing. That was the year Auxein Corporation was granted permission to spray unregulated amounts of monosodium glutamate combined with MfG from other sources on agricultural products. We learned of this by accident when in 1999 I read of the approval of AuxiGro WP Metabolic Primer (AuxiGro) and the free glutamic acid used in AuxiGro, in the Federal Register.

The story of AuxiGro is the story of a double-blind study you won't hear from the glutamate people. In the late 1990s, one of our MSG-sensitive friends reported that she'd eaten potatoes in addition to her otherwise standard diet, and had an MSG reaction. Another friend independently told the same story, but his reaction had been to head lettuce. What did Jack and I believe? Our friends had gone off the deep end. That's what we believed. Maybe too much MSG had gotten to them.

Then came the information that MSG was being sprayed on crops. Two of the crops that had been used in field tests and then brought to market (prior to approval) were head lettuce and potatoes. Our small sample double-blind study told us that monosodium glutamate sprayed on crops could cause adverse reactions in MSG-sensitive people.

The EPA regulates (or fails to regulate) the use of pesticide products. As you might have anticipated, we brought the information we had on the toxic effects of MSG to the EPA, where, after being given politically correct lip service, it was ignored.

In August 2001, we finally had the opportunity to file a formal objection to the EPA's approval of AuxiGro. The original approval had been granted before we knew it had been requested. The second application was a modification of the original application, and we could object to it.

As might have been anticipated, our efforts were fruitless. We were advised the EPA had submitted our data to AuxiGro's producer, and had been informed that the data we'd submitted to the FDA were meaningless. Even anticipating that this was the kind of response we'd get from the federal government each time we challenged the safety of MfG in general or monosodium glutamate in particular, we never passed up an opportunity that might give us a foot in the door to exposing MfG's toxic potential.

Auxein Corporation had also applied to the State of California for approval of its product, AuxiGro, and the glutamic acid contained in it. California often has more stringent environmental standards than other states or even the federal government, so registration of AuxiGro there would be of great value to Auxein Corporation's investors. In May 1999, the California Department of Food and Agriculture (CDFA) approved spraying MSG on wine grapes (calling the spray a fertilizer). Steven Wong, Branch Chief, Agricultural Commodities and Regulatory Services, told us that to have a product approved for use as a fertilizer in California, a company had to do little more than make application.

In April 2000, and again in July 2001, the California Department of Pesticide Regulation (CDPR) approved spraying MSG on wine grapes (calling it a fungicide). Barry Cortez, Branch Chief, CDPR, told us the CDPR would only turn down a product if it appeared to be ineffective, and AuxiGro didn't appear to be ineffective. Oh, the power of industry! Registration of an effective poison wouldn't necessarily be turned down.

Other approvals followed until the MSG in AuxiGro was approved for use on all agricultural commodities.

Discussion with the CDPR was more protracted than discussion with the EPA, but the end result was the same. California chose to allow use of unregulated amounts of MfG for agricultural purposes. It wasn't called monosodium glutamate, hydrolyzed protein, or MSG, however. In the approvals it was called L-glutamic acid — but make no mistake, it was manufactured free L-glutamic acid complete with its impurities.

We first formally presented details of our displeasure to the CDPR on June 8, 1999. We didn't know at the time that the glutamate industry had as much clout with the CDPR as it had with agencies of the federal government.

Because we were early on the scene in California, we were able to track the progress of AuxiGro's approval. As we challenged it, the CDPR turned to authorities on the subject of amino acid safety, not to Taylor and Ebert — that would have been too obvious — but to their friends and colleagues on the faculty of the University of California at Davis. UC Davis is a school with a well-deserved great reputation in the field of food technology, where Food Science and Technology faculty are members of the Institute for Food Technologists (IFT), where Taylor and Ebert serve as role models.

Despite our protests, processed free glutamic acid was ultimately approved for use in pesticide products in California.

We'd repeatedly asked the CDPR questions, which if answered, would have jeopardized the approval of AuxiGro and "L-glutamic acid." They were simple but possibly embarrassing questions such as:

> "How, and by what company, is the processed free glutamic acid used in AuxiGro produced? Is it produced by Ajinomoto or others by a method of bacterial fermentation wherein '...bacteria...excrete glutamic acid

they synthesize outside of their cell membrane into
[a liquid nutrient] medium and accumulate there?
The glutamic acid is separated from the fermentation
broth by filtration, concentration, acidification, and
crystallization...'?"

A little bird had told us that the "L-glutamic acid" used in AuxiGro
was monosodium glutamate imported from Germany.

The Truth in Labeling Campaign asked the CDPR how a proper
scientific evaluation could be made without having the answers to
those questions. Had the CDPR responded, its answer would have
been that a proper scientific evaluation couldn't be made without this
information. In fact, a proper scientific evaluation hadn't been done. But
that question was one of many that CDPR Branch Chief Barry Cortez
refused to answer.

Auxein Corporation, later known as Emerald BioAgriculture, also
applied to the National Organic Standards Board (NOSB) for organic
certification, with the independently owned and operated Organic
Materials Review Institute (OMRI) pushing for its approval. When Jack
made his presentation to the NOSB, the OMRI report recommending
approval was already in the hands of NOSB board members. I really
do believe that only because of Jack's presentation, which included
demonstration of the fact that AuxiGro was a synthetic product, did the
board deny approval of AuxiGro and L-glutamic acid for use as organics.

OMRI

When the NOSB rejected the application, we assumed OMRI would
cancel its relationship with AuxiGro. We found, however, that OMRI
merely tabled the issue, suggesting to us that they would try again
sometime in the future to have AuxiGro approved for use as an organic.

In subsequent discussions with OMRI, Jack mentioned that fertilizers
like hydrolyzed fish protein were also synthetic, and could cause adverse
reactions in some MSG-sensitive people. The OMRI person became
combative, declaring that he'd observed production of the fish protein,
and all the producer did was take the remains of fish and grind them up
for use as a fertilizer. As Jack pushed him to review the entire process, he
finally admitted that they pour "a little enzyme" into the mixture. Thus,

he confirmed there was MfG in the hydrolyzed fish protein: protein (in fish) combined with acids or enzymes ("a little enzyme") creates MfG.

During the course of various discussions, we learned that OMRI charged a fee for reviewing a product and recommending that it be added to the NOSB list of approved organic products. We also learned that if a product was approved, the producing company would pay OMRI an annual fee as long as it remained approved. If there was no NOSB approval, there'd be no annual fees paid to OMRI. It sure looked like a conflict of interest to us.

Use of AuxiGro has not been limited to the United States. We saw notice in the early 2000's that Intrachem had been licensed to distribute AuxiGro in Europe.

At the end of the decade, registration of AuxiGro in the US lapsed. We found that AuxiGro had failed to apply for reregistration with either the EPA or the CDPR, and therefore, could no longer be legally sold in the United States. That may have changed, but whether used in the U.S. or not, AuxiGro is now being offered for sale throughout the world.

Interestingly, the withdrawal of AuxiGro from the American market coincided with the attention being given to the strange disappearance of bees from bee hives, referred to as "Bee Disappearance Disorder." Jack was interested in the phenomenon, and found that the disorder had spread beyond the boundaries of the United States, and began to occur in other countries.

Being familiar with the glutamate literature, and recognizing that scientists had found that laboratory animals lost their way in mazes after being exposed to MSG, it occurred to Jack that bees visiting plants that had been sprayed with MSG (in AuxiGro) might become disoriented, fail to find their way back to their hives, and die. At the time of the onset of the Bee Disappearance Disorder, AuxiGro was often sprayed from crop dusting airplanes. It appeared obvious that bees would be exposed to AuxiGro sprayed in this fashion both at the time of spraying and through residues that would remain on plants. Thus, spraying MSG on growing crops might be contributing to the disappearance of bees. That idea was reinforced by the knowledge that many MSG sensitive people become disoriented following ingestion of MSG in amounts that exceeded their tolerance levels.

Jack made a number of attempts to discuss his theory with people in the bee industry and related agencies. To my knowledge, it never received attention from any industry organization, agency, or person, although there has been discussion of the possibility that bee disappearance disorder was caused by pesticides. I cannot help but wonder if Emerald BioAgriculture found that the bee disappearance was actually linked to use of AuxiGro.

The fact that AuxiGro was being offered for sale around the world meant nothing until 2003, when we found that Italian and Spanish wines labeled 2003 and after were no longer safe for Jack to drink. He had been having MSG reactions to most California wines since wine made with grapes sprayed with AuxiGro had come to market, but had been drinking European wine without a problem.

Eventually we discovered that AuxiGro was being distributed throughout Europe (Spain, Italy, Portugal, and Switzerland), Asia, Latin America, and Canada if not elsewhere. Details of its distribution were secret. We attempted to question Intrachem Bio International SA, Geneva, Switzerland, the AuxiGro distributor for at least parts of Europe, but they refused to respond to our questions. By 2011, Jack could not tolerate certain wines from Italy, Spain, Chile, France, and Argentina. On the other hand, he could generally tolerate California wines from small and/or organic vineyards.

NAET

By the end of 1999, Jack was sure the end of his life was just around the corner. He was miserable. He simply never felt well. One day when I was out doing whatever I was doing, Jack decided to stop at a health fair at the county fairgrounds not far from our home. Jack didn't know what he thought he'd do there, but he evidently had nothing better to do.

As he walked, Jack came upon a chiropractor with a portable computer talking to people about diagnosing and then treating their allergies. For $15, he could select a list of products that included many he knew to contain MSG, be tested for sensitivity to them, and be told to which ones he was allergic or sensitive.

After watching the chiropractor conduct tests on a number of people, he decided to give the man $15 to run through one of his panels, and was amazed to find the man was totally correct in identifying foods to which Jack knew he'd react.

The chiropractor had come to the health fair to encourage people to come to his office for Nambudripad's Allergy Elimination Technique (NAET) treatments. Jack was tempted to try NAET, but had seen NAET demonstrated years before, and had been totally unimpressed. Then, too, this chiropractor made Jack uncomfortable.

I was home when Jack returned from the health fair, and recounted his experience. Then Jack told me something I already knew: he had nothing to lose. He wanted to believe that the NAET treatments could help him. He wouldn't have admitted it, even to himself, but he was in such a state that I think he might have tried anything.

I understood Jack was desperate. I didn't find fault with his interest in NAET, but made two recommendations. First, he should get the opinion of a Chinese medicine doctor who had helped him at one time, and was now helping me. Second, I insisted that if he decided to start the NAET program, he should go to the person who'd invented it instead of one of her students. I reasoned that if he went to the local chiropractor, whom he really didn't care for, and the program didn't help him, he'd never know if it was the chiropractor or NAET itself that didn't work for him.

Jack started NAET treatments in January 2000. Both the theory and the procedure are simple and straightforward. An allergy/sensitivity, as defined in NAET terms, is a blockage to the flow of energy caused by an offending substance. In NAET, the channels of energy flow (the meridians) are held open through the use of acupuncture or acupressure while the offending substance is held in the patient's hand, and the energy of the offending substance begins to flow unencumbered from meridian to meridian. Once the energy of the offending substance has passed through all the meridians (approximately 24-25 hours), the blockage will usually have been eliminated, i.e., the allergy/sensitivity will have been resolved. On occasion, it will take more than one treatment to resolve a sensitivity.

Dr. Devi Nambudripad, who had developed NAET, was very clear in her instructions. NAET would clear blockages to the flow of energy, so she was certain it could help Jack, but it wouldn't cure his sensitivity to MSG, since MSG was a toxin, a poison, and NAET wouldn't protect him from that. Nambudripad told him that while NAET could help him avoid the immediate reactions — what most people would call "allergic reactions" — it couldn't prevent the addition of toxins to his body. She warned him not to be complacent and eat food that contained MSG just because he no longer had what others might call an allergic reaction to it.

It was immediately clear that if the system worked at all, it was going to take Jack considerable time to clear all his energy blockages. The energy of MSG in the ingredient known as monosodium glutamate might differ from the energy of what we were still calling MSG in sodium caseinate, for example, and each might have to be addressed separately. Therefore, Jack began to drive the 60 miles to Buena Park three or four times a week to progress as quickly as he could. Sometimes I would go with him, and eventually I began to use NAET for my own assorted allergies.

A couple of years into treatment, we met two women who'd seen Nambudripad in England, and were so grateful for her help, that when problems arose, they traveled from England to see her in California. We'd been using muscle testing much as a chiropractor would to detect allergies and sensitivities, but muscle testing done in this manner required a person to test you, and was awkward to do in public. These women introduced us to the O-ring tester; showed us how to use it at home and in the grocery store; and taught us how to use the O-ring tester to scan a menu not only for the selection of food, but to identify foods that were safe to eat. The O-ring tester is nothing more than a spring attached to a dial that moves when the spring is depressed. It's a kinesiology device to test muscle strength that can be used by a single person. If it really worked as the ladies described, it would be the ultimate in protection, and Jack might never have an MSG attack again.

MORE TRAVEL

Toward the end of April, Jack and I set off again for France. This time, we spent three days dining in Paris, then rented a car and drove east through Metz and Nancy to Strasbourg, stopping at Sarrebourg, home of Mephisto shoes, and from there on to Alsace and a self-guided tour of its cheese factories and vineyards. We headed south to Colmar and Illhaeussann for dinner at its world-class restaurant, Auberge de L'ill, and journeyed to Mulhouse and the incredible collection at the National

Auto Museum of France. We then drove back west and north to Paris and more exceptional food.

Throughout our trip, the French seemed to be using more processed food than previously, but Jack found it easy to avoid. The NAET treatments may have been helping him avoid allergic-type reactions, but there was no way for him to know that. He was not yet using the O-ring tester.

In late September 2000, Jack was privileged to address the annual meeting of the Celiac Sprue Association. People with Celiac Sprue, a genetic disease that results in malabsorption of grains, have some of the same problems with food labels that MSG-sensitive people have. Grains are often hidden in food under names other than wheat, rye, barley or oats.

On this trip, Jack had his first test of the efficacy of NAET treatments. He went to a restaurant he was sure used processed foods, and after eating food for which he'd already been treated, sat at the table waiting to become seriously ill — but nothing happened. NAET had been validated.

In October 2000, Jack traveled to India with the Chicago Council on Foreign Relations. He didn't yet know of the O-ring tester, but managed pretty well to avoid MfG. He did make one stupid mistake, however; he succumbed to some freshly made ice cream, forgetting that milk was likely loaded with parasites, and came down with explosive diarrhea.

In 2003, we rented a car and traveled through Spain. Jack had discovered Paradors, where the finest food was served. Eating in Paradors posed no problem. Everywhere else, he had to be more vigilant because the use of processed food was growing. At that time, the Glutamate Association and the IGTC had a presence in Europe in the person of the comité des fabricants d'acide glutamique de la CEE [Committee of Glutamic Acid Manufacturers of the European Economic Community] (COFAG), which had offices in Paris.

By this time, Jack was using the O-ring tester religiously to test food, and doing very well with it. He hadn't yet grown to believe he could use it to read a menu, so every once-in-a-while he inadvertently ordered something he couldn't eat. I was very good about ordering something Jack would enjoy eating if the meal he'd ordered didn't work for him.

In February 2004, we rented a car in New Zealand and spent three weeks touring both islands. Jack had gone to Antarctica some years earlier with a number of environmentalists, all of whom lived in New Zealand. From discussions with them, it appeared New Zealand had to be the safest place for him to travel with respect to environmental problems and food purity.

In planning our three-week trip, we tried to pack lightly, and as part of that program, Jack bought cotton disposable underwear. He put on his first pair of disposable underwear the day we caught the plane to New Zealand, and continued to wear it through the day of our arrival and into the evening, when our hotel room became available.

The following morning, Jack found he was passing blood when he urinated, and with each urination, the amount of blood he passed became greater.

We considered the options: go to a local hospital or return to the U.S. It was doubtful Jack was having a reaction to MSG, because he'd brought his own food on the airplane, and eaten carefully once in Auckland. It was possible, of course, that he was simply having an allergic reaction to something other than MSG, a possibility that had begun presenting itself from time to time. A physician friend had said it wasn't uncommon for someone with an allergy or sensitivity to a specific substance to develop secondary ones, as the first one would have weakened the body's defenses against other allergies and sensitivities. This time-dependent sensitization, which might be thought of as a progressive increase in the size of a response over repeated exposure to a substance, is referred to as kindling.

It was time to ask questions. What had Jack eaten that was different, or what was he doing that he didn't do at home? The only thing we could think of was the disposable underwear.

By this time, both Jack and I were comfortable using kinesiology, so I used it to question what was causing the bleeding. Muscle-strength testing told us that Jack was unable to tolerate the spandex band in the disposable underwear, and that the spandex band had brought on the bleeding.

Jack changed to his regular underwear (I had insisted on bringing two pair) and by the next morning, the bleeding had stopped. We purchased new underwear, for the rest of the trip, and the bleeding became history.

But there were other problems. It had become our practice to stop during the first day in any new town at a local grocery store, and Auckland was no exception. Jack was shocked to find that with the exception of a row of organic chickens, all the chickens in the rows and rows of them in the counter had been injected with some kind of basting material containing MSG. Chicken was thereby eliminated from Jack's food choices.

Jack had no problem avoiding chicken, but New Zealand wasn't agreeing with him. Would you believe that quality New Zealand olive oil infused with lemon was causing him a problem? In discussing the virtues of olive oil with a gentleman selling it at an open-air market, we learned that in lemon-infused olive oil, lemons are cut up and left sitting in oil for a time sufficient to allow the acid in the lemons to break down any protein present in the oil, producing "just a little" free glutamic acid (MfG). The restaurants we'd gone to, in their efforts to provide high-quality meals, used the more sophisticated and expensive lemon-infused olive oil. Once Jack made that discovery, he made certain that olive oil he used in restaurants was olive oil, only, and he was fine.

Even after eliminating chicken and lemon-infused olive oil from his diet, he found it difficult to eat in New Zealand. It was the generosity of the people that was doing him in. A simple cookie came surrounded by whipped cream that contained MfG. These kind people just couldn't understand that when Jack asked for a hamburger with nothing else on the plate, other things they might put on my plate might be bad for him. People there just couldn't bring themselves to give Jack something they considered less than the best they had to offer.

By 2005, life had become routine. Jack was using the O-ring tester. He bought nothing and ate nothing without first testing it with either the O-ring or simple arm testing. Eating in restaurants became possible again as long as he could find places that could provide him with fresh, unprocessed food. He rarely ate at the homes of family or friends for fear he might have a reaction while with them, but there were a few who'd make meals without using anything processed, and he really appreciated that.

A VISIT TO THE EMERGENCY ROOM

Jack's first visit as a patient to a hospital (outside of when he was born) took place in the wee hours of the morning of July 12, 2005. Our granddaughter Hannah, had come for a two-week vacation, as was our custom for grandchildren who reached the ripe old age of 10. On the evening of July 11, we'd gone to the Pageant of the Masters in Laguna Beach, an extraordinary presentation of classical works of art populated by real people within frames and backgrounds designed for them. We had dinner at one of our favorite restaurants, enjoyed the presentation, and were on the way home when Jack said he was feeling worse than not well. I suggested we stop at the hospital we'd be passing, but Jack chose not to do that. (I wasn't driving.)

Three hours later, Jack was having chest pain and such difficulty breathing that he woke me, who in turn woke Hannah, and Jack let me drive him to the hospital. Friends have remarked that Jack must have been in truly bad condition if he didn't insist on driving himself.

I had Hannah dress for the occasion, and later remarked that her pajamas might have been a better choice. I brought a pillow and blanket for Hannah, and Hannah (a voracious reader) brought enough books to see her through the night. I expressed great concern over Jack's condition, but Hannah was blasé about the whole thing. She had brothers, she told us, and had been in emergency rooms many times.

In the end, it was determined only that Jack was fibrillating, but because a heart attack couldn't be ruled out, he'd be kept in the hospital for a day or two for observation. By morning, he was feeling no pain, and had no trouble communicating. Actually, he never had trouble communicating, even in the wee hours of the morning before. So Hannah and I brought him a cooler loaded with ice and food to take him through the day, stayed to chat for a half hour, and then took off for Disneyland. We'd purchased Disneyland passes for the three of us for two days each, which meant the two of us could spend an extra day at Disney without additional charge. But before we set out each day, we brought Jack a new ice chest and a day's supply of food.

Jack was very well cared for in the hospital. The nurses offered to make whatever food he might be able to eat, a hardboiled egg, for example. They seemed to have no difficulty understanding the extent of his sensitivity. Similarly, the physicians respected the fact that binders and fillers in pills that might have been prescribed probably wouldn't be tolerated, so they didn't prescribe any.

Jack was hooked up to a cardiac monitor and monitored with the rest of the patients in the cardiac care unit. The technician told him that in all his years, he'd not seen as interesting a heartbeat. When he'd come in, Jack had been fibrillating, but that had stopped. Now Jack was told he was fibrillating again.

On the second night, while sleeping, Jack's heartbeat evidently deteriorated. He was awakened by someone shaking him and was surprised to find eight people surrounding his bed.

His heartbeat must have improved after he was awakened, because they provided no intervention while his fibrillation continued. The next day, after stressing it on a treadmill, his heart resumed a normal beat, and the cardiologist dismissed him from the hospital. The cardiologist assured Jack he'd not had a heart attack, and he didn't know what else he could do for him. Once home, Jack began fibrillating again — and continued fibrillating for five days. That's not uncommon timing for fibrillation following MfG ingestion.

When Jack left the hospital, he convinced the nurse to give him a sample of the heart monitor contacts that had been glued to his chest. I still have some. They were Red Dot contacts produced by 3M. He'd asked for the sample because as they removed the contacts from his chest, he observed that the center of each contact that had touched his skin had a small bulb of gelatinous material. He knew that the glue on the contact likely contained some starch, an ingredient that would have small amounts of MfG, but didn't think such a small amount would cause such an immediate reaction. After the contacts were removed, he realized there would also have been MfG in the gelatin that had made contact with his skin.

Back home, Jack contacted 3M, told them of his situation, and asked for a list of the ingredients used in the Red Dot product. They refused, stating the information was proprietary. Jack then called a friend who was a major 3M customer, and asked for his help in getting the ingredient list. It turned out that it was the guar gum in the gelatinous material that was the offending ingredient. The 3M laboratory had found a small amount of free glutamic acid in the guar gum, which a representative claimed in a carefully worded e-mail, was so very small that it wouldn't have caused his reaction. I wish I had $10 for each time I've heard someone say that the amount of MSG was so small Jack couldn't have reacted to it.

Given Jack's experience, he considered it appropriate to ask 3M to disclose in the Red Dot product insert the fact that MfG-sensitive people with little tolerance for MfG might experience a reaction from the product. 3M refused.

TRAVEL

We traveled to Portugal and Barcelona in September 2006, flying United Airlines to Barcelona through Madrid, then on to the Guggenheim Museum in Bilbao, and on to Lisbon. It was morning when we arrived in Barcelona without luggage — which, we were told, had not been sent on from Madrid. Uncomfortable as the lack of clean clothes might have been, the real problem lay in the fact that Jack had packed his blood pressure medicine in one of the suitcases that was lost, and the exact formulation he needed (without MfG in its binders and fillers) wasn't available in either Spain or Portugal.

From Federal Express, we also learned that neither Spain nor Portugal could accept medication from outside the country. We tried a hospital, a compounding pharmacy and the American Consulate, without success. Finally, some kind person, who shall remain nameless, told us of a small country in Europe with pharmacies that could accomplish extraordinary things. Jack's blood pressure medicine came from France, where it was made, and arrived in two days. (Incidentally, it cost far less coming from France via another country to Portugal than it would have cost Jack in the U.S.)

As the years went by despite more MfG being poured into processed food, and a growing number of wines Jack could no longer tolerate, he was using the O-ring tester to choose restaurants and scan menus for safe foods, and rarely suffered a reaction. Santa Fe and the Santa Fe Opera were favorites of ours. We also spent two weeks in Berlin and three weeks in Italy in 2007 and 2009. Kinesiology relies on energy, not on language, so menus written in foreign languages never presented a problem.

KUNIO TORRII

In mid-March, 2008, the financial magazine *Forbes* published "The MSG Cure," but the only thing it might have been a cure for was Ajinomoto's pocketbook. It was an interview with Kunio Torii, evidently "the highest-ranking scientist at Ajinomoto," presenting a whole new spin on the hype designed to draw the consumers' attention from the fact that MSG (and MfG), in any form, cause brain lesions, endocrine disorders, and adverse reactions such as asthma and migraine headache. In short, its intent was to convince readers that monosodium glutamate is "safe." In the interview, Torii talked of feeding monosodium glutamate as a "cure" to the people most vulnerable to its toxic effects — the very young, those who are ill, and the elderly — the people most likely to have compromised blood-brain barriers and peripheral glutamate receptors being stressed.

That's too sick to be a sick joke.

THE BERKELEY WELLNESS LETTER

The Berkeley Wellness Letter remained a reliable source of glutamate industry misinformation. Every couple of years, it published an article that gives every indication of having been written by the Glutes, spinning the tale that MSG is safe. The last industry-friendly MSG article we saw before Jack died was "The ABCs of MSG" in September 2009.

From conversations I had with people at Berkeley, I concluded that a group that did newsletters for a number of organizations was writing the Berkeley Wellness Letter. I'd concluded that no one on its editorial staff had written the article, which was likely written by someone at the IGTC or its agent, the IFIC.

SENOMYX

On April 5, 2005, an article by Melanie Warner in the *New York Times* had talked of a new biotechnology company called Senomyx. This company had developed a product in the laboratory that would replicate the flavor enhancing attributes of monosodium glutamate.

The article gave every indication that the product would act neurologically through the taste buds (glutamate receptors) just like monosodium glutamate does. The company indicated that neither the name Senomyx, nor the chemical compound used in Senomyx would be listed on ingredient labels. Instead, Senomyx would be included as one of the undisclosed ingredients in "artificial flavors." Flavors, by law, are considered proprietary ingredients, so food companies aren't required to disclose the names of ingredients contained in them.

In the article, the chief executive of Senomyx was quoted as stating that its organization was helping companies clean up their labels. Clean labels are labels for ingredients that contain toxic substances but give no clue to that fact.

Following the announcement that Senomyx had an MSG replacement that wouldn't have to be disclosed on food labels, Kraft Foods, Nestle, Coca Cola, and Campbell's put up $30,000,000 to assist the company in its product development in exchange for the rights to use the ingredients in certain types of foods and beverages.

One of the selling points made to investors was the claim that the amount of Senomyx to be used in any food product would be so small that it wouldn't require FDA approval. That led us to believe the product had been developed using the relatively new process of nanotechnology, which offers many benefits to industry, but is untested for safety in foods. I, and others, have great concern that the minute particles produced by nanotechnology can easily pass through the intestinal wall, placenta, and blood-brain barrier. And there's nothing to say otherwise.

Not long after its introduction, the Senomyx product received safety approval from the Flavor and Extract Manufacturers Association (FEMA). That's how it's done in the food industry. The company or companies producing or using a product declare they've found it to be GRAS (generally recognized as safe). They have, or claim to have, research that demonstrates the product is safe. From that point, the spin masters use the industry's declaration of GRAS to sell stock, encourage venture capital investments, and market their product to consumers — without mentioning the fact that it had not been declared GRAS by the FDA.

In the case of the Senomyx monosodium glutamate replacement product, the safety study on which the FEMA-GRAS approval was based was a three-month study that was never published nor made available to those who asked FEMA for it. I've seen articles that indicate that FEMA is a government agency, but that's not true. FEMA is a non-profit agency, funded by and for the benefit of companies in the flavor and extract industries.

Over the years, I've repeatedly asked the FDA why pharmaceutical firms spend over $100 million dollars and take more than seven years to have a pharmaceutical approved for marketing, while Senomyx is able to put a product made in a laboratory and arbitrarily referred to as food on the market essentially without testing for safety. I haven't yet received a reply.

A number of companies joined the bandwagon to license and use Senomyx's MSG replacement. Worldwide distribution was divided, with Nestle controlling an area that included Europe, while Ajinomoto had a territory that included Asia and the U.S.

In mid-2010, some of the biggest names in Big Food, including Kraft, Campbell's and Nestle, announced they'd be cutting the use of salt in their products by a minimum of 20 percent. That coincided with the FDA's announcement that it might soon require the reduction of salt in processed foods. That coincidence reminded me of another that just happened to benefit big business. Quite some time ago, Jack alerted the FDA to the fact that there was benzene in the adhesive products used to secure dentures. Nine months later, the fact that there had been benzene in denture products was disclosed to the public. It was only announced after manufacturers had replaced all the denture products containing benzene.

In 2018 Senomyx was acquired by Firmenich, the "world's largest privately owned perfume and taste company," based in Switzerland. Firmenich manufactures numerous flavoring ingredients for processed foods including one called "savoury modifier 80," described by the company as being a "powerful ingredient providing great umami taste…"

The fact that Senomyx is no longer in business makes little difference in the scheme of things as similar, if not exactly identical additives are being manufactured. The Flavor and Extract Manufacturers Association is still labeling them GRAS (FEMA GRAS), and to our knowledge none have been tested for safety or analyzed by the FDA.

Chapter Twelve

Where Were We as 2011 Ended?

It was November 2011. It had been 20-plus years since Jack and Dr. Schwartz had gone to Washington. Some of the glutamate industry players we'd met in the 1990s had changed. New dirty tricks had been added to Big Food's playbook, but there was no threat to industry that MSG/MfG would have to be identified on the labels of the products that contained it. And there was even less chance that there might be a warning about the presence of MfG.

When I checked recently, David Hattan and Linda Tollefson were still at the FDA, while Richard Ronk, Walter Glinsmann, and Fred Shank had moved on. With Monsanto's Michael Taylor serving as President Obama's FDA Deputy Commissioner for Foods, however, there could be no question that the FDA would continue to represent industry as opposed to consumers.

As far as MSG activity was concerned, there wasn't much to monitor. I watched the research put out by the glutes, and invariably wrote critiques when their work was published in medical or nutrition journals that would accept letters to the editors. Some of my letters had been published, but many had not. It's not for lack of knowledge or writing skill that my letters had been rejected. In recent years, glutamate industry interests had assumed an increasingly greater presence in medical/nutritional publishing.

Much of the work that the glutes passed off as research now consisted of reports of seminars and workshops during which industry-sponsored researchers sat around tables discussing the virtues of MSG. The rest came from publication of papers claiming the existence of a fifth taste sensation (the taste of monosodium glutamate), which they referred to as umami.

In the first half of the 20th century, monosodium glutamate was characterized as a "white, almost odorless, crystalline powder with a slightly sweet or salty taste[193]. Early encyclopedia definitions of monosodium glutamate (which was said to contain glutamic acid, sodium, moisture, and not more than one percent impurities) described it as an essentially tasteless substance. What's more, most MSG-sensitive people (who'd love to be able to detect the taste of MSG and thereby avoid ingesting it) claimed there's no taste to monosodium glutamate. Could it be, then, that umami is little more than a clever contrivance/device/public relations effort to draw attention away from the fact that MSG is toxic and help legitimize its use? A Japanese word for "delicious," this adjective umami is being groomed to substitute for the term "monosodium glutamate," which is increasingly being recognized as synonymous with the adjective "toxic."

Umami" appears to be one of the glutamate industry's many attempts to pair pleasant sounding words with "monosodium glutamate," with no concern as to whether the way in which the words are used makes any sense.

Fifth taste or not, MSG/umami is toxic. As Shakespeare might have said, umami is a tale told by an idiot, full of sound and fury, signifying nothing — it's a fairy tale that's been sold to the American public. In my humble opinion, there is no "fifth taste," and the perception of one is the perception of glutamate-receptors firing.

Attempts to work with relevant government agencies have proved fruitless. We've scrutinized their activities and seen no hint of change. Similarly, it's obvious that Congress is in the pocket of the glutamate industry — there's no other explanation for its inaction — so any energy we might have spent trying to educate its members would have been largely wasted.

You may have seen one of the many reports of young athletes dropping on the playing field and dying from heart attacks. Since Jack knew that protein powders and power drinks — which are loaded with free glutamic acid and free aspartic acid — are actively marketed to young athletes, he spent considerable time and energy attempting to contact athletes who have suffered ventricular fibrillation. His goal was simply to alert the athletic community to the fact that MSG/MfG can cause heart irregularities, and that extreme physical stress combined with MfG will exacerbate what might otherwise be a mild MfG/aspartame reaction.

I had retired from full-time focus on MSG. I knew where MfG was hidden in food.

Hidden Sources of MfG

Ingredients that *always* contain MfG

Glutamic acid (E 620) *1	Calcium caseinate,	Soy protein isolate
Glutamate (E 620)	Sodium caseinate	anything "Protein"
Monosodium glutamate	Yeast extract, Torula yeast	anything "Protein fortified"
(E 621)	Yeast food, Yeast nutrient,	anything "Protein concentrate"
Monopotassium glutamate	Nutritional yeast	anything "Protein isolate"
(E 622)	Autolyzed yeast,	Zinc proteinate
Calcium glutamate (E 623)	Brewer's yeast	anything "Proteinate"
Monoammonium glutamate	Gelatin	Soy sauce
(E 624)	Textured protein	Soy sauce extract
Magnesium glutamate	Whey protein	Protease
(E 625)	Whey protein concentrate	anything "Enzyme modified"
Natrium glutamate	Whey protein isolate	anything containing "Enzymes"
anything "Hydrolyzed"	Soy protein	anything "Fermented"
any "Hydrolyzed protein"	Soy protein concentrate	Vetsin
		Ajinomoto

Ingredients that often contain or produce MfG during processing

Carrageenan (E 407)	Maltodextrin	Malted barley
Bouillon and broth	Oligodextrin	Pectin (E 440)
Stock	Citric acid, Citrate (E 330)	Malt extract
any "Flavors" or "flavoring"	anything "Ultra-pasteurized"	Seasonings
Natural flavor	Barley malt	Soy milk

Ingredients suspected of containing or creating sufficient processed free glutamic acid to serve as MfG-reaction triggers in HIGHLY SENSITIVE people

Corn starch	Milk powder	Vinegar
Corn syrup	Reduced fat milk (skim; 1%; 2%)	Balsamic vinegar
Modified food starch	most things "Low fat" or "No fat"	certain Amino Acid Chelates
Lipolyzed butter fat	anything "Enriched"	(Citrate, Aspartate, and
Dextrose	anything "Vitamin enriched"	Glutamate are used as
Rice syrup	anything "Pasteurized"	chelating agents with mineral
Brown rice syrup	Annatto	supplements.)

*1 E numbers are use in Europe in place of food additive names.

I knew how the Glutes engineer their research to come to the predetermined conclusion that MSG is safe. There was little for me to do besides keep up the website, Facebook pages, and blogs through which we provide honest information about MSG/MfG to those who might benefit from it.

Jack had handled most of the questions that came through e-mails and phone calls, and when the opportunity arose, he'd give an interview. That, in itself, took a major portion of his day.

Much of the rest of Jack's day was given to grocery shopping and cooking. When he had been forced to retire, he'd taken up cooking, becoming an outstanding cook.

We hadn't seen anything from Andrew Ebert lately. I'd guessed he was still drawing a salary, being invaluable to the industry. After all, the man has a network of friends in places like the AMA, ADA, WHO and EU, and his golf games with friends in those places wouldn't make the headlines. In July 2011, I saw a piece on the IFT Food Additives website indicating that Ebert was chair of the Food Chemical Codex Food Ingredients' Expert Committee.

Steve Taylor, longtime spokesperson for the glutamate industry, was still an IFT member, and still served as director of The Food Allergy Research and Resource Program (FARRP), which, according to the program of the IFT's 2011 Annual Meeting and Food Expo, fills a distinct void in the area of allergenic foods. "FARRP is a 14-year partnership between food industry and the University of Nebraska employing comprehensive, sound and thorough approaches to food safety.... FARRP offers training, workshops and consultation on processing issues and regulatory aspects of allergenic foods and food ingredients, has an extensive food allergy database and works with leading researchers to improve the safety of food products globally." Taylor's bio didn't mention MSG or that Ajinomoto and/or the IGTC are his other employers.

Every once in a while, an intrepid researcher completed a study that demonstrated MSG is toxic. But even if the researcher found a journal to publish the study, there would be virtually no mention of it in major media. Michael Hermanussen and Ka He are among the names you won't see.

The misinformation spewed forth by the industry remained unchallenged:

- The FDA/industry has continued to claim that the glutamic acid found intact in protein is identical to manufactured free glutamic acid, ignoring the fact that when amino acids are freed from protein, impurities (not present in intact protein) are invariably produced.

- As "proof" that its products are safe, the glutamate industry points to studies in which the number of subjects who reacted to monosodium glutamate was roughly the same as the number of subjects who reacted to a placebo that contains hydrolyzed protein products, autolyzed yeast, other MfG-containing ingredients, and/or aspartame. "Fail to confirm..." is the terminology they used. Moreover, while the industry's friends at the FDA accepted these badly flawed studies as proof of the safety of MSG, consumer reports of adverse reactions following ingestion of MSG were dismissed as anecdotal.

- The FDA/industry has continued to claim that just a little bit of MSG won't hurt anyone. (The fact that just a little bit of peanut can kill a peanut-sensitive child isn't considered.)

- The FDA/industry has continued to claim that MSG reactions are mild and transitory, occurring within two hours after its ingestion. Research that says otherwise is ignored.

The dirty tricks have continued, some in new or slightly modified form.

Every now and then, an obvious glutamate industry-sponsored person (often a "student") e-mails the Truth in Labeling Campaign for the purpose, it would seem, of provoking a fight. Jack always answered questions truthfully and was careful not to say anything that might be taken out of context and somehow be used to discredit him. He was always careful to note that he was pleased to share what he had learned over the years, but that he was not a physician.

The best trick, if it was a dirty trick, was played by Ted and Melissa. I had hired them to redo our website, which was in serious need of renovation. They agreed on financial arrangements in fall 2010, and began redesigning the site a couple of months later. They were to give it a new look and install a new navigation system, but leave the text largely as it was. I would approve each piece of the package they presented as they moved along.

For a couple months, Ted, Melissa, and I worked comfortably together. Then, in an unexplainable turnaround, Ted and Melissa began telling me what I was to do and when I was supposed to produce the work they needed to move forward. They also began to demand payment, which they had previously agreed would be made when the site was completed.

Frustrated, and unable to get more than inappropriate demands from Ted and Melissa, I determined to take the problem to arbitration as stipulated in their original contract. Would you believe the address needed to have arbitration papers served in San Diego County couldn't be found? Even the address on file with the state related to the incorporation of Ted and Melissa's company turned out to be false.

I was able to find Melissa on the Internet. Her family lived in the San Diego area, but she didn't seem to live with them. Melissa took college courses in San Diego, too, but the school wouldn't give me an address.

Ted was more difficult to trace. In surfing the web, however, using clues I had picked up in various conversations, I found a picture of Ted and a description of the work he'd done at the University of Wisconsin — but the name attributed to the face was Ted Durkee not Ted Bradley, the name by which I'd known him.

Dirty trick? Maybe not. This couple was to collect a couple thousand dollars at the end of the project. They'd worked with me amiably up to a point, and then the atmosphere had changed. Do I know for a certainty that this was a dirty trick? No, I don't, but I can't imagine this young couple would give up a couple thousand dollars and leave us in the lurch for no reason at all.

Confusion seems to be an ongoing goal of the glutamate industry. We were, therefore, suspicious when a group called "Citizens to Label Genetically Engineered Food" changed its name to "Truth in Labeling Coalition" and engaged in fundraising.

We knew there were agents of the glutamate industry who pretended to be concerned about the toxic effects of MSG. These people were building reputations as being concerned about MSG toxicity, but when the glutamate industry starts its next offensive, they'll invariably declare to their readers, web followers, and the media that they made a mistake in saying there was need to be concerned about adverse reactions from MSG. They'll say to all who'll listen that MSG is safe. Or they'll say that it would be great if the FDA would require labeling all products that contain more than 3 grams of MSG. You might think of them as double agents, being paid by one side only.

Were our phones still bugged, if they ever were? Maybe yes, maybe no. I doubt we maintain threat status with the glutamate industry. But I know that bugging us — our phones, houses, cars, computers, and things I haven't even thought of — wouldn't be a drop in their anti-exposure bucket. Ajinomoto Co., Inc., is a multi-billion-dollar company. It's still true today.

We were proud of our accomplishments, few though they may be. Awareness of the toxic potential of MSG was growing and continues to grow. Not growing enough, but growing. Our website, our Facebook pages, and our blogs were helping MSG-sensitive people understand MSG's toxic potential and avoid it. We've never made a penny from all we've done, but we've earned the respect of those we've been able to help by minimizing their reactions to MSG, and their notes of thanks have been payment enough.

We understood that kinesiology can be used as a tool by people who are sensitive to MSG (or any other chemical) to warn them against consuming food, pharmaceuticals, or dietary supplements that contain it. We've continued to share that information, and the FDA hasn't yet figured out a way to prevent consumers from using that knowledge.

We were cognizant of things that still needed attention.

Not all MfG in processed food was identified on product labels. Only "monosodium glutamate," one of more than 40 common MfG-containing ingredients, gives even a clue to the presence of MfG.

Instead of being banned, AuxiGro went international. Interchem (and possibly other distributors) began distributing it worldwide.

As 2011 ended it became increasingly difficult for Jack to eat. For all intents and purposes, anything made with wine was made with grapes sprayed with AuxiGro. Therefore, if an Italian, French, or Spanish restaurant prepared dishes with wine or used wine sauces, chances were Jack wouldn't be able to tolerate them.

We'd learned a great deal on this journey. Possibly the saddest was the fact that all too many people willingly sacrifice principles for money.

Included are the people who go on and on about pure foods and preventive medicine — talking the good talk about avoiding MSG while personally profiting from sales of dietary supplements with binders and fillers that contain neurotoxic MSG and/or neurotoxic aspartic acid, and sales of protein drinks that contain neurotoxic MfG, neurotoxic aspartic acid (as in aspartame), and neurotoxic L-cysteine.

Chapter Thirteen

Ten Years Later

January 2012, and Jack was gone. The people he had helped with MSG toxicity were on their own to defend themselves against the onslaught of excitotoxic amino acids being poured into food in ever increasing amounts.

I had lots to think about. Would I stay in California? I had a grand five-bedroom house on a hill overlooking Rancho Santa Fe where I'd lived with Jack for 25 years. Knowing that Jack could never survive a hospital and nursing home, we'd built two bedrooms onto the original house so live-in help would be comfortable if we ever had the need. Would I stay?

I'd certainly continue writing. I knew I would, because that's who I am. And it didn't occur to me to stop telling people that MSG is toxic – that the free glutamate in MSG is toxic. To tell the world that free glutamate is hidden in processed food, where free glutamate is hidden in processed food, who's behind hiding excitotoxic amino acids in processed food — and that the FDA makes it all possible.

But I also had to put the pieces of my life back together. Probably the single most significant event in the long road to recovery was a chance encounter I had early on with a perfect stranger in the Apple Computer store in Encinitas, California. We were seated at a large rectangular table, where my vocal admiration for the beautiful display on her computer screen transformed itself into a recitation about anxiety that was making it difficult for me to use the computer properly, which in turn led to her suggestion that I **must** take the Mindfulness Based Stress Reduction Course given at Scripps Hospital in Encinitas.

The guilt for not having done more to save Jack had to go. The memories of marvelous people and the wonderful times had to replace the memories of violent mood swings, Jack's fear of dying, and the violent death he suffered as his nervous system seemed to explode. I'm still working on it.

I would pick up writing from where I'd left off in 2012 when Jack lost his battle against glutamate toxicity. First, I'd add the names of new ingredients designed to better hide MfG in processed foods. That would be easy, as I'd updated the list of hidden sources of MfG each time a new name surfaced.

But there was more I would do. I never really thought about it. Yes, I would write as I always had. But Jack and I were a team, he speaking out while I wrote. And after the trauma of saying goodbye had passed, I somehow knew that speaking the truth, as hard as speaking might be for me, would be something I would do. I didn't think about it, it just happened.

I would start by exposing lies. I would try to master Facebook and Twitter, and maybe even sign up for LinkedIn, although in the past I had avoided social media like the plague.

Lies told to promote MSG and its excitotoxic component MfG as harmless food additives hadn't changed much since Ajinomoto set up its MSG-is-safe-shop (the International Glutamate Technical Committee — IGTC) in 1969. And if consumers understood Ajinomoto's lies, there would be no question about the dangers posed by ingestion of MSG and MfG.

Before 1989, we believed what Ajinomoto wanted us to believe: monosodium glutamate is a functional flavor enhancer with no side effects. We knew Jack reacted to the substance and he wasn't the only one to do so, but we still had no idea there were many others like him. We believed that only a few people reacted to monosodium glutamate; that aside from Jack, their reactions were mild and transitory, and it would take 5 grams of MSG to cause a reaction.

By the end of 1989, however, we were starting to consider that not everything we heard from the glutamate industry was true. But we didn't yet understand that the Glutes were systematically laying down the foundation for their web of deception.

On the one hand, they built a scenario of simple lies, like "MSG has been used safely for over 1,000 years," and "the glutamate in MSG is identical to the glutamate in plants and animals, including humans."

Those simple lies, still in play today, appear to be aimed at deceiving consumers along with influencing media and regulators.

But more important to their success in hiding the toxicity of MSG/MfG would be their success in keeping scientists and government regulators from **even thinking** about the fact that MfG is a neurotransmitter, which would activate glutamate receptors in the mouth and tongue, and if taken in sufficient quantity, would kill brain cells by causing glutamate receptors in the mouth and tongue to fire repeatedly until their targeted glutamate receptors died.

When discussing the actions of MfG and possible unwanted reactions, the subject of ingestion and digestion of MfG would be covered in considerable detail by the Glutes, while the subject of glutamate receptors in the mouth and on the tongue being stimulated and overstimulated would be systematically ignored.

Following is the essence of the story the Glutes created and continue to repeat over and over again to represent the activity of MSG. This is the scenario they not only pushed, but pushed to the exclusion of all others — the "digestion scenario."

> A person eats a protein containing glutamate that 1) proceeds through normal digestion; 2) is released from the protein in which it is bound; 3) enters the bloodstream, and 4) proceeds to the brain. There, we are told, if substantial amounts of glutamate accumulate (glutamate, which having been digested is now **free** glutamate), it may cause brain damage. But, the Glutes will tell you, it is highly unlikely that enough glutamate will accumulate to cause brain damage. And that, they claim, proves that ingestion of glutamate does not cause either brain damage or adverse reactions.

You may disagree with the conclusions, but the premise is basically true. Glutamate bound in protein that is ingested, digested, and passed from the blood to the brain will probably not cause brain damage.

But that leaves unexplained how someone who ate something with MSG/MfG in it would **instantaneously** have a migraine headache or go into anaphylactic shock. I had observed those instant reactions with Jack.

And there was no way that such an immediate reaction to MSG could have been triggered by glutamate going the lengthy route from food to blood to brain.

It took a while, but the bits and pieces of what I knew about MfG eventually glued themselves together. Glutamate has many functions, and multi-tasking is its specialty. It is a building block of protein, present in most every cell in the body. It is a neurotransmitter, a "chemical messenger" essential to sending messages between nerve cells.

It is also a neurotoxic (brain damaging) amino acid. When present in well-regulated amounts, it enables the brain to function properly. But when accumulated in excess in interstitial tissue (areas between cells), glutamate becomes an excitotoxic neurotransmitter firing repeatedly until its targeted glutamate receptors die.

When glutamate that is found outside of protein (free glutamate) is taken into the mouth, two things happen. One, some is ingested with everything else that is ingested, moving down the esophagus into the stomach and intestines where it undergoes digestion, is taken into the bloodstream, and as needed, is taken into the brain.

At the same time, other free glutamate will activate glutamate receptors in the mouth and on the tongue. This is free glutamate acting as a neurotransmitter. Some might think of these receptors as taste buds, which some of them are, but regardless, each is the first in a string of nerve fibers that transmit chemical messages to nerves in various parts of your body.

Glutamate neurotransmitters are made up of strings of nerve cells and are stored in thin-walled membrane sacs called synaptic vesicles, located at the end of each nerve cell. Each vesicle can contain thousands of neurotransmitter molecules.

As a message or signal travels along a nerve cell toward the next nerve cell it will contact, the electrical charge of the signal causes the vesicles of glutamate neurotransmitters to release their contents into a fluid-filled space that's between nerve cells. This space is called a synapse. On the other side of the synapse is the next nerve cell. Glutamate must bind to specific message-receiving receptors on this next nerve cell. After binding, glutamate then triggers a change or action in this next nerve cell, and the communication signal continues on its way from nerve cell to nerve cell.

How glutamate acts at the synapse between nerve cells can either strengthen or weaken the communication signal between these cells, which then affects the function to be carried out. Less than the right amount of glutamate released at the right places for the right amount of time results in poor "communication." Too much glutamate can damage cells.

That, in fact, is what happens when more glutamate than is needed for normal body function (taken in its free form) enters the mouth. That will often happen when ultra-processed foods that are loaded with glutamate-containing flavor enhancers and fake proteins (such as Just Egg and Beyond Meat) are consumed. What alone would be a harmless neurotransmitter, when joined by a quantity of other glutamate molecules, becomes part of an army of excitotoxic neurotransmitters killing brain cells.

Jack's reaction to MfG/MfG was a reaction caused by a neurotoxic neurotransmitter in the central, or possibly the peripheral, nervous system, not by anything related to blood circulation or digestion.

I don't pretend to understand the science of it all, but what transpires when free glutamate enters the mouth can be easily visualized in the graphic below.

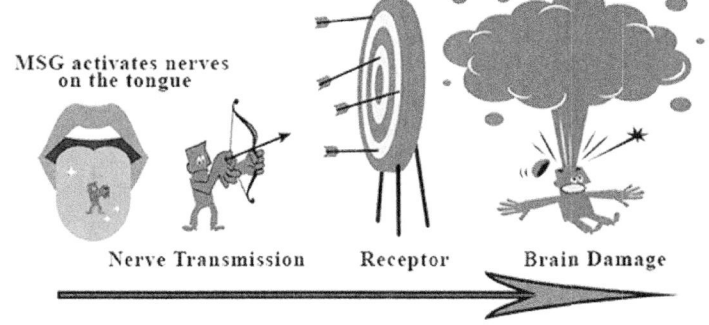

MSG activates nerves on the tongue

Nerve Transmission   Receptor   Brain Damage

It wasn't until 2012 that I began to realize that the picture painted by the Glutes of how MSG was handled by humans wasn't just a simple lie. It was the very foundation of the web of distraction they were spinning. Not a lie in one sense of the word, but an invention that would draw you away from the truth, having greater impact than any simple lie could have.

Lies didn't change much after Jack died. What changed was that people were beginning to question the lies.

Since 1968, there had been reports of brain damage, endocrine disorders, and adverse reactions following ingestion of MSG. A May 3-5, 1998 NIH-sponsored conference titled *The Glutamate Cascade: Common Pathways of Central Nervous System Disease States*, explored the evidence that glutamate appeared to be associated with several seemingly diverse disease processes of the central nervous system (CNS)[194]. Disorders in which a role for glutamate had already been demonstrated included: addiction (tolerance, sensitization, dependence, and/or neurotoxicity that is associated with certain drugs including opiates, cocaine, amphetamine, alcohol), stroke, epilepsy, brain trauma, certain types of neuropathic pain, AIDS dementia, schizophrenia, depression, anxiety, and dementia/Alzheimer's.

Today a search of the National Library of Medicine's PubMed.gov includes considerably more.

Before I wrote and published "The toxicity/safety of processed free glutamic acid (MSG): a study in suppression of information," I had read of FDA-industry cooperation/collusion in a number of books, including:

Eating May Be Hazardous To Your Health — The Case Against Food Additives, by Jacqueline Verrett and Jean Carper

Health at Gunpoint: The FDA's Silent War Against Health Freedom, by James Gormley

The Rise Of Tyranny, by Jonathan W. Emord

Codex Alimentarius Global Food Imperialism by Scott Tips

Inside the FDA: The Business and Politics Behind the Drugs We Take and the Food We Eat, by Fran Hawthorne

Stolen Harvest: The Hijacking of the Global Food Supply,

by Vandana Shiva

The Truth about the Drug Companies: How They Deceive Us and What to Do about It, by Marcia Angell

I had no idea of how extensive and deep-seated that collusion really was until I began researching the subject for "Industry's FDA."

Industry's FDA

The FDA's cooperation with Ajinomoto to promote the use of monosodium glutamate (MSG) was first evidenced in 1969 during testimony given before the Senate Select Committee on Nutrition and Health on the safety of MSG by then FDA Commissioner Ley. Commissioner Ley testified to four studies that allegedly demonstrated the safety of MSG. It was later confirmed that two of those studies had not been completed, and the others didn't exist.

Since that time FDA/industry cooperation has included:

- Telling blatant lies about the safety of MSG, lies originating with the glutamate industry and repeated by the FDA.
- Dispensing complementary information about MSG while withholding information that might be considered negative.
- Officially approving study protocols for MSG-is-safe studies that used placebos known to cause the same reactions as those caused by MSG test material.
- Allowing glutamate-industry propaganda to be displayed on the FDA webpage https://www.fda.gov/food/food-additives-petitions/questions-and-answers-monosodium-glutamate-msg
- Refusing to collect reports of reactions to MSG "because we know that no one reacts to MSG."

(You'll find more about Industry's FDA in Appendix I. It's worth reading.)

We hadn't doubted that there were authoritative bodies that concluded that MSG was a harmless flavor enhancer, but hadn't realized that all had received study materials from Ajinomoto and its agents, and none had done independent research. We only learned that when Jack, sitting next to a perfect stranger on an airplane, heard the story of her participation in a review of the safety of MSG conducted by one of the Glutes "authoritative bodies." Regulators and/or authoritative bodies cited by the glutamate industry as "authoritative bodies" did no research of their own, but were given copies of FDA opinions on MSG safety or were provided review information by Ajinomoto, its not-for-profit corporations, and/or its agents — the International Food Information Council (IFIC) and the International Life Sciences Institute (ILSI), for example. And the vast body of published research demonstrating monosodium glutamate toxicity was never shown to them.

One of the Glutes most often repeated lies is that MSG is very well researched and has been found safe by "authoritative" bodies or "well respected international agencies."

We couldn't understand how glutamate in MSG could cause adverse reactions while glutamate in a lamb chop didn't, until we came across the 1994 research of Rundlett and Armstrong[12]. They demonstrated that processed food containing free L-glutamic acid invariably contained free D-glutamic acid. And with that knowledge, we were able to search out information about the various impurities found in monosodium glutamate and the other ingredients that contained MfG.

Possibly the most regularly regurgitated lie told by the Glutes is the lie that glutamate contained in MSG is identical to glutamate in the human body. The research of Rundlett and Armstrong exposed that for the lie it is.

Actually, glutamate in the human body is L-glutamate — L-glutamate only, whereas any manufactured glutamate (found in monosodium glutamate and pea protein isolate, for example) is made up of both L-glutamate, D-glutamate, and other impurities.

Impurities include D-glutamic acid, pyroglutamic acid, and other impurities depending on the starting materials used (or materials used to feed the genetically modified bacteria) and the extent of processing.

Glutamate metabolism is another popular subject. My own research was key to understanding that there was no evidence that metabolism of MSG yields the same effects as metabolism of whole protein. Search for such evidence simply failed to uncover any.

Two whoppers that Ajinomoto has been pushing lately are "MSG is naturally made, similar to yogurt, vinegar and wine," and "monosodium glutamate occurs naturally in food." Actually, MSG in the U.S. is manufactured using genetically modified bacteria that excrete glutamic acid through their cell walls. The only similarity to yogurt, vinegar, and wine is that their production includes fermentation. And MSG is manufactured. In the United States, monosodium glutamate is produced in Ajinomoto's plant in Eddyville, Iowa. It doesn't occur naturally in anything.

Sometimes the claim is made that MSG is safe because the FDA has given it GRAS (generally recognized as safe) status. Actually, the FDA relies on industry to determine what products are "safe." Only when products are undeniably toxic or are not produced by Big Food or Big Pharma will the FDA deem them unsafe. The FDA does not order drug recalls, regardless of evidence of toxicity, unless directed to do so by Big Pharma. The FDA does no recalls on food or other non-drug items. If things were to get hot, so to speak, the FDA would orchestrate a voluntary recall to be done by the manufacturer.

Evidence of glutamate industry/FDA collusion, in effect since 1968 if not before, attests to the FDA's conflict of interest.

THE SUPER LIE

The biggest lie of them all, of course, is that MfG is harmless. But it's more than a lie. It's not just that MfG is harmful. MfG is the perfect poison.

MARKETING THE LIES

Glutamate industry marketing has always been interesting as well as clever. When there was evidence that that the safety of MSG was being questioned, as there was in 1975, the Glutes had the FDA convene a review of the safety of MSG. The FDA's conclusion, which was interpreted by the Glutes as finding that MSG was "safe," seemed to take care of that situation.

In the years leading up to 1993, as the safety of MSG was again being vigorously questioned, the Glutes had the FDA convene another review of the safety of MSG. Again, after the Glutes rejected the FDA's initial report, the FDA produced a new one.

But after 2010, something evidently wasn't going as planned. You won't find them admitting it, but sales of MSG were slipping. Maybe the webpages of The Truth in Labeling Campaign were getting attention. Maybe our social media pages were having an impact. Clearly, paramedics and emergency-room physicians had begun to recognize MSG reactions. Or maybe it was from one mom cautioning another that she shouldn't feed her kid MSG. But something wasn't going as planned by the Glutes, and they've been advertising up a storm to make up for it.

The most persuasive of advertising agencies have nothing on the glutamate industry's advertising prowess. A key element in their attack on the truth is to pair feel-good words and phrases with monosodium glutamate and repeat that pairing over and over and over again. That gets the victim in the right frame of mind. On top of that are the endorsements of "experts" and celebrities, listing the virtues of MSG (low salt, makes food taste better), lies about things that aren't easy to check out (there's MSG in tomatoes), and degrading remarks about those who have opposing opinions. Racist and xenophobia are words being bandied about as this is being written. Brainwashing is what it all boils down to.

LIES OF A DIFFERENT SORT

Perhaps they're not lies in the traditional sense, but inventing fictions that draw the consumer's attention away from the truth for the purpose of promoting a toxic product fits with my understanding of a lie.

...THE FIFTH TASTE

Years ago, Ajinomoto began to work on convincing the public that MSG had a taste of its own, a fifth taste along with sweet, sour, salty, and bitter. What a genius way to justify the use of MSG. No matter that for years monosodium glutamate had been recognized as a food additive that had no taste of its own but something that enhanced the flavor of food with which it was paired. No matter that MSG-sensitive people, who would have loved to recognize the "taste" of MSG so they could avoid it, maintain they can't taste it.

...UMAMI

Then came the brilliant idea that the word "delicious," which is "umami" in Japanese, should be substituted for the term "monosodium glutamate," which was becoming increasingly unpopular. And "umami" began to be (and still is) vigorously marketed.

But that still wasn't doing the trick. Better that MSG should be sold as something more than an additive that makes food taste better. Better to market MSG to save the environment, to reduce sodium intake, and to increase plants/crops production. Then from time to time, depending on the audience, stimulating appetite would be added as an advantage of MSG ingestion, particularly for the sick and for the elderly.

The fact that excitotoxic (brain damaging) glutamic acid was the active ingredient in MSG was, of course, overlooked.

..."PLANT-BASED FOODS"

With growing awareness of the need to produce goods in a more environmentally friendly way, so-called "plant-based" meat and/or protein substitutes are being promoted as "healthy," eco-conscious choices. Sadly, what Big Food advertises as "plant-based" is really chemical based, concocted from toxic chemicals derived from plants. Often the only "plants" involved in "plant-based" proteins are the chemical plants they're produced in.

"Meat substitutes" is another way you may have heard these concoctions described. Their relevance to the discussion here is that in producing what they refer to as proteins, they have taken protein from plants and broken it down into its constituent amino acids: excitotoxic (brain damaging) glutamic acid, and excitotoxic aspartic acid. And the average consumer won't have a clue.

...LOW SALT

Then there's the promotion vigorously supported by the FDA to reduce salt intake — regardless of whether or not you as an individual need to do so. The Glutes (with the blessings of the FDA) have one or more campaigns going to get people to substitute MSG for table salt. The fact that MSG contains excitotoxic (brain damaging) glutamic acid and aspartic acid is never mentioned.

...PLANT GROWTH ENHANCERS

It's too early to know if it will be ongoing, but there's also a campaign to use MSG as a fertilizer.

When used as a fertilizer, MSG will not only stimulate plant growth but will find its way into the fruit, grain, or vegetable produced by the plant to which it is applied. AuxiGro WP Metabolic Primer, the first MSG-laced plant "growth enhancer" we know of to hit the market, was approved for spraying on every crop we know of, with no restrictions on the amount of MfG that might remain in and/or on crops when brought to market. Even before consumers had an inkling that crops were being sprayed, the Truth in Labeling Campaign received reports that MSG-sensitive consumers had gotten sick from head lettuce and potatoes — two crops that the EPA had been approved for experimental (and undisclosed) use of AuxiGro.

CELEBRITIES TO LURE YOU

And as in all good advertising, spokespersons are of the utmost importance. Luminaries of all sorts are valuable, but celebrity chefs are the best when it comes to marketing something you're going to eat. The Glutes' celeb chefs include Andrew Zimmern, David Chang, Chris Koetke (Dean of the Sun Valley Culinary Institute), and restaurateurs Grant Achatz, Michael Anthony, Alexander Bourdas, David Kinch, and Adam Fleischman (Umami Burger chain founder).

ENDORSEMENTS

The last time we looked at The Glutamate Association's msgfacts.com page, the "authoritative bodies" they had convinced to endorse the safety of MSG included:

- Food Standards Australia New Zealand (FSANZ);

- The Joint Expert Committee on Food Additives (JECFA) of the United Nations Food and Agriculture Organization;

- World Health Organization (WHO), and

- The European Community's (EC) Scientific Committee for Foods

One of the Glutes' favorites over time has been the assertion that "other authoritative bodies" have found MSG to be safe. One such organization was Helen Keller International. They were supplementing monosodium glutamate with vitamin A in Indonesia to counteract xerophthalmia, an eye disease caused by lack of vitamin A. Helen Keller International didn't consider that to be an endorsement of the safety of MSG, nor had they considered the toxic potential of MSG. They were not pleased to learn their name was being used in this manner.

THE BASIC TRUTH

On the flip side of every lie, rests the face of truth. Jack has been gone for ten years, and in that time, I determined that while each lie is interesting and adds something to the deceptive and misleading dialog of the glutamate industry, there are really only five essential truths about toxic MSG.

1) Monosodium glutamate (MSG) is always manufactured.

No matter how produced, monosodium glutamate is composed of three ingredients, sodium, glutamic acid and moisture, along with impurities that are the inevitable result of manufacture.

2) The toxic ingredient/component in MSG is its manufactured free glutamic acid (MfG).

- Glutamate, whether manufactured or not, is an excitotoxic amino acid, meaning that when present in tightly regulated amounts, it will be found in cells where it serves as a building block of protein, and as a neurotransmitter sending signals from glutamate stimuli to glutamate receptors throughout the body. But when accumulated outside of cells in quantities greater than needed for normal body function, neurotransmitter MfG becomes excitotoxic, firing repeatedly at receptor cells until the cells at which it is firing die.

- MfG is a free amino acid.

- MfG remains an excitotoxic chemical regardless of the names of ingredients that contain it.

- MfG is a component of all flavor-enhancing ingredients and all protein substitutes.

- There are more than 40 ingredients known to contain MfG.

3) MfG becomes toxic only when it accumulates in amounts greater than are needed for normal body function.

Glutamate bound in protein, in an unadulterated steak or tomato, for example, does not contribute to excitotoxicity.

While the amount of MfG found in any one ingredient may be insufficient to cause excitotoxicity, since production of MfG was "modernized" in 1957, there has been more than enough MfG to cause excitotoxicity if more than one processed or ultra-processed ingredient is consumed during the course of a day. Ultra-processed food will always contain MfG to make up for the flavor lost by using poor quality produce and chemicals.

Having had time to myself that I had not had in years, and reaping the benefits of mindfulness practice, I began to understand things I had seen before but not noticed. I could see the studies in my mind's eye — solid evidence from studies published in medical journals. The MfG that caused brain damage followed by obesity in Olney's mice also causes brain damage followed by obesity in humans.

4) Excitotoxic MfG ingested by pregnant females and passed to their fetuses over the placenta will cause brain damage in the area of the arcuate nucleus of the hypothalamus of the fetus that would have regulated appetite and satiety had it not been obliterated by MSG.

5) MfG is the perfect poison.

PROPAGANDA

According to the Merriam-Webster dictionary, propaganda is the spreading of ideas, information, or rumor for the purpose of helping or injuring an institution, a cause or a person. And Ajinomoto has made an art — no holds barred — of producing the most elaborate fiction alleging that MSG is a harmless food or food additive. Leaving nothing to chance, it has garnered the support of authoritative bodies to testify to the truth of their lies, invoked the name of science, and employed the finest wordsmiths to seduce the public into believing them. My blogs often focus on their propaganda.

MACULAR DEGENERATION

From studies published in medical journals, it is clear that glutamate plays a significant role in headaches, asthma, diabetes, muscle pain, atrial fibrillation, ischemia, trauma, seizures, stroke, Alzheimer's disease, amyotrophic lateral sclerosis (ALS), Huntington's disease, Parkinson's disease, depression, multiple sclerosis, schizophrenia, obsessive compulsive disorder (OCD), epilepsy, addiction, attention deficit/hyperactivity disorder (ADHD), frontotemporal dementia and autism.

It is also clear that glutamate toxicity plays a significant role in obesity, infertility and macular degeneration. While the subject of glutamate-induced obesity has been discussed here in considerable detail, the subjects of infertility and macular degeneration have not.

In 1957, Brandon Lucas and Ian Newhouse[194] first noticed that severe retinal lesions could be produced in suckling mice (and to some extent in adult mice) by a single injection of glutamate. Studies confirming their findings using neonatal rodents[195-198] and adult rabbits[199] followed shortly, with others being reported from time to time[200-205]. These studies concerned themselves not only with the confirmation of monosodium glutamate-induced retinal lesions, but with the formulation and testing of hypotheses to explain the phenomenon.

In 2002, Ohguro et al.[206] found that rats fed 10 grams of sodium glutamate (97.5 percent sodium glutamate and 2.5 percent sodium ribonucleotide) added to a 100 gram daily diet for as little as three months had a significant increase in amount of glutamic acid in viteous, had damage to the renina and deficits in retinal function.

Ohguro et al. also documented the cumulative effect of damage caused by daily ingestion of MSG.

Other reports of toxic effects of monosodium glutamate have come from studies at the University of Pecs, Hungary[207-208].

On May 31, 2022, I found 566 citations at pubmed.com (a search at the National Library of Medicine) for the combination of "glutamate" and "retinal degeneration."

INFERTILITY

In the 1970s it was demonstrated by Olney and others that reproductive dysfunction follows glutamate-induced brain lesions in the arcuate nucleus of the hypothalamus (AN), and that monosodium glutamate fed to laboratory animals was an excellent source of free glutamate.

Indeed, reproductive dysfunction can be caused by excitotoxic amino acids ingested by pregnant and nursing women and delivered to fetuses and newborns who exhibit infertility as they reach maturity.

The onset of the infertility crisis can be traced to the introduction of excessive amounts of MfG being made available to humans following the modernization of MSG manufacture in 1957.

ADVERSE REACTIONS

In addition to the brain damage caused by ingestion of MfG, there are glutamate-induced adverse reactions such as fibromyalgia, asthma, and heart irregularities. We began compiling lists in the early 1990s — lists that have grown as we were able to verify reports we were given. The following table was up-to-date at the time this book was published.

Adverse reactions known to be caused from time to time by MfG

Cardiac	Neurological	Respiratory
Arrhythmia	Depression	Asthma
Atrial fibrillation	Mood swings	Shortness of breath
Tachycardia...	Rage reactions	Chest pain
Rapid heartbeat,	Migraine headache	Tightness in the chest
Palpitations	Dizziness	Runny nose
Slow heartbeat	Light-headedness	Sneezing
Angina	Loss of balance	
Extreme rise or drop	Disorientation	**Urological / Genital**
in blood pressure	Mental confusion	
	Anxiety	Swelling of the prostate
Circulatory	Panic attacks	Swelling of the vagina
	Hyperactivity	Vaginal spotting
Swelling	Behavioral problems	Frequent urination
	in children	Nocturia
Gastrointestinal	Attention deficit disorders	
	Lethargy	**Skin**
Diarrhea Nausea/vomiting	Sleepiness	
Stomach cramps	Insomnia	Hives (both internal and
Irritable bowel	Numbness or paralysis	external)
Swelling of hemorrhoids	Seizures	Rash
and/or anus area	Sciatica	Mouth lesions
Rectal bleeding	Slurred speech	Temporary tightness or
Bloating	Chills and shakes	partial paralysis
	Shuddering	(numbness or tingling)
Muscular	Tinnitus	of the skin
		Flushing
Flu-like achiness	**Visual**	Extreme dryness of
Joint pain		the mouth
Stiffness	Blurred vision	Face swelling
	Difficulty focusing	Tongue swelling
	Pressure around eyes	Bags under eyes

Early on we recognized that these adverse reactions bear a remarkable resemblance to the lists of possible side effects you'll find in prescription drug inserts. And that makes sense, because free glutamate is, in fact, a neurological drug that also happens to be used in food.

KNOW WHERE YOUR INFORMATION IS COMING FROM

If you're going to protect yourself and your loved ones, you have to know how the Glutes operate.

Start with the FDA. Most Americans still believe that the folks at the FDA are looking out for their welfare. Just consider that as this is being written, the FDA has refused for 19 months to respond to a Citizen Petition to remove MSG and MfG from its GRAS (generally recognized as safe) list, and has ignored requests for information submitted under the Freedom of Information Act. If that doesn't convince concerned citizens of FDA/industry collusion, reading "Industry's FDA," (Appendix I) should do the trick.

Then there are the news sources. Not since the 1991 *60 Minutes* program on MSG has any major media outlet dared say anything that might even suggest that MSG is anything less than a safe food additive.

And all media outlets carry MSG-is-safe propaganda, including big names such as *The Washington Post, Canadian Broadcasting Company,* and *The New York Times.*

Medical schools don't teach their students to screen for MSG or MfG toxicity, and physicians often refer a suspected MSG sensitivity to an allergist who won't recognize it for what it is because a reaction to MfG is a reaction to a poison, not an allergic reaction. Researchers in the U.S. can't get grants to support studies of MSG toxicity. And medical journals don't publish studies that find MSG to have toxic potential. That's how it's been for a long time and how it still is.

THE DIFFICULT CONCEPT OF EXCITOTOXICITY

Prior to 1957, when Ajinomoto retooled the manufacture of MSG, flooding the market with virtually unlimited amounts of MfG, the word "excitotoxicity" would not have been found in the dictionary.

Similarly, prior to 1957, there had been no unexplained increases in obesity, infertility, autism, multiple sclerosis, or neurodegenerative disease.

But all that changed in 1957, the year that mass-production of MSG was introduced, Lucas and Newhouse studying retinal degeneration found that sodium L-glutamate, as well as a number of other materials, damaged the retina of albino mice. In 1969, Olney demonstrated that monosodium glutamate killed brain cells in the arcuate nucleus of the hypothalamus, at which time, it was demonstrated that glutamate-induced brain damage to the arcuate nucleus of the hypothalamus of neonatal animals was followed by obesity, reproductive dysfunction, behavioral disturbances and more[140].

When consumed in controlled quantities, glutamate is essential to normal body function as a neurotransmitter and building block of protein. But when consumed in excess, in quantities greater than needed for normal body function, it becomes excitotoxic, firing repeatedly and killing its targeted glutamate receptors. Olney coined the term "excitotoxin" in 1969 to describe the actions of glutamic acid which had been delivered in monosodium glutamate (MSG)[140]. At the time, researchers were administering glutamate to laboratory animals subcutaneously using Accent brand MSG because it had been observed that MSG was as effective for inflicting brain damage as more expensive pharmaceutical grade L-glutamate[140].

These are the stories I tell daily on blogs, Facebook, and Twitter. These are the stories I send to newspapers, TV news outlets, magazines, and medical journals — all of which are under industry pressure to ignore anything that suggests that MSG and MfG are anything other than safe.

Chapter Fourteen

The Obesity Epidemic

This could have been the end of the story — bringing the book up to date in 2022. But as I put Jack's papers in order and cleaned out my office, I began thinking again about the brain damage, obesity and reproductive dysfunction that Olney and others had observed, and pondered on how that would express itself in humans. After all, if MfG was causing silent brain damage, there's no way we would know it.

Review of Olney's research had raised a question and I couldn't let it go: Might excitotoxic glutamate fed to immature humans also result in uncontrollable obesity? And might that largely account for the obesity **epidemic**? The timing looked just right. I was curious.

In 1969, Olney demonstrated that glutamic acid fed in quantity to immature animals causes lesions in the arcuate nucleus of the hypothalamus, resulting in gross obesity as the animals matured. Although lost cells were replaced, they were not replaced with neurons. The neurons that might have regulated food intake were gone.

Olney's subjects were infant animals. Newborn humans and fetuses would be comparable. Both have immature brains that are vulnerable to damage caused by excitotoxic glutamate.

Olney fed exceedingly large amount of glutamate to those animals. Since 1957, exceedingly large amounts of free glutamate have been available, accessible and consumed by humans.

In 1957, the method for producing glutamate was changed to facilitate virtually unlimited production of free glutamate and MSG. And ultra-processed foods, which contain flavor-enhancing free glutamate in ingredients such as autolyzed yeast extract, sodium caseinate, maltodextrin, glutamic acid, and hydrolyzed proteins as well as MSG, became readily available, accessible, and increasingly more popular.

The glutamate delivered to Olney's neonatal animals was delivered in food fed to them. The glutamate delivered to humans with vulnerable brains is delivered by their pregnant or nursing mothers.

Newborn humans can only receive glutamate in mothers' milk or infant formula. But fetuses are "fed" through the umbilical cord and through the placenta. And if a pregnant woman ingested large quantities of free glutamate, as she might if her diet included processed and ultra-processed food, the excitotoxic free glutamate would cause damage to the brain of her fetus just as it caused damage to the brains of Olney's animals.

How might ingestion of free glutamate by a pregnant woman relate to the obesity **epidemic?** There was no obesity epidemic prior to 1957. The obesity epidemic was established after virtually unlimited amounts of excitotoxic glutamate became readily available, accessible, and consumed in processed and ultra-processed food. The obesity **epidemic** grew as growing numbers of children who had been "fed" MfG as fetuses by their pregnant mothers were born.

Intractable human obesity is:

- produced in a fetus by MfG that a pregnant woman consumes and then "delivers" to her fetus,

- not caused by lack of will power, laziness, or genetic deficiency, and

- something over which a person has no control.

My work with glutamate-induced obesity won't be finished until those who suffer from uncontrollable weight problems understand that they are not to blame for being unable to control an uncontrollable condition. And until women understand that ingestion of large quantities of free glutamate while pregnant will damage the brains of their unborn children.

That won't be easy by any means, for it appears that obesity has become an industry, with industrial giants unwilling to give up pieces of their cash cow. The 2015 article in the March 24 *Atlantic* by Harriet Brown, "How Obesity Became a Disease — And, as a consequence, how weight loss became an industry"[195] and her book, *Body of Truth*[196] cover that subject.

Is there any other way to explain the fact that *Obesity*, the journal of The Obesity Society, has refused to discuss the idea that intractable obesity might be caused by glutamate-induced brain damage caused by excitotoxic free glutamate "fed" to fetuses by pregnant women? Or the fact that letters to The Obesity Society's CEO, Anthony G. Comuzzie, have gone unanswered?

Chapter Fifteen

The Perfect Poison

B eing a mystery buff, it occurred to me long ago that excitotoxic glutamic acid and aspartic acid are the perfect poisons. Both are amino acids found naturally in the human body. Both play vital roles in maintaining normal body function and will occur as normal constituents of the human diet.

What's the perfect poison? A webpage on the subject of undetected murder suggested that whatever is used to do the deed should be undetectable at autopsy. And MSG can't be topped for that. Glutamate will be found in virtually every cell in the human body. There's also glutamate in the protein that you eat. To begin with, today no one would suspect that glutamate could or would be used as a poison. But even if suspected, there would be no way for an autopsy to determine that the deceased had more than normal amounts of glutamate in their bodies.

Epilogue

When I was young, I lived in a middle-class world of wonder and privilege. I sneaked a peek at the half-nude African natives in my father's *National Geographic* magazines, but read nothing of their hardships. I traveled through the southern U.S. and saw signs that said "No Blacks" and "No Jews," but we, who were Jews, always had a place to stay so those signs meant nothing to me. I was born in a hospital and lived in a brick two-story house with my brother, sister, parents, and housekeeper. My father belonged to a country club. I knew nothing of the millions of others who didn't have such things.

With Jack's disability, a whole new world came into focus. Before I came to know the people who were purposely pouring toxins into our food supply, I couldn't understand why it was that Catholic friends would go to confession, and why, every year on Yom Kippur, we were given the opportunity, and indeed urged, to repent for our sins. Once we were introduced to people like Hattan and his colleagues at the FDA and their friends at The Glutamate Association and the IGTC, I began to understand the role of confession as it was being used by the dishonest, unethical, and/or immoral people who transgress, confess, and transgress again. I became aware of a whole world of people for whom dishonesty was a way of life — confession or not.

When I was an undergraduate, I worked 20 hours a week in Northwestern University's psychology department, running experiments for faculty members. As a graduate student, I became a research assistant, again doing research for faculty members. Research as I knew it involved finding answers to questions to add to a particular field's knowledge base.

Following Jack's disability, I learned the world of research had changed. There were, to be sure, researchers searching for answers to add to the base of knowledge, but there were also those who turned out reports to prove whatever their handlers demanded of them. It was hard enough to accept the fact that my colleagues would take employment with companies that required them to prostitute themselves, but there were others who held positions at colleges and universities. And medical schools! The schools themselves gave these so-called researchers permission to use their facilities for a fee referred to as "overhead."

The University of Iowa was the first such institution I encountered. A cadre of researchers led by Dr. Lloyd Filer, Mead-Johnson Professor in the Department of Pediatrics, claimed their research demonstrated that both monosodium glutamate and aspartame were harmless food additives.

Today, I know what I saw in 1989-1990 was just the tip of the iceberg. Today, the air we breathe, the earth that sustains the bulk of our food supply, the water that sustains what's left of the aquatic population, and the water we're given to drink are all polluted, and that pollution is ongoing and growing. Much that's done in the name of moderating the effects of that pollution consists of applying toxic chemicals to air, earth and water.

Today, universities like the University of California at Davis are turning out scores of food technologists, some of whom make their livings inventing novel ways to substitute chemicals for foods, as cost-cutting measures. MSG and aspartame are the products I know best. Both contain neurotoxic amino acids that cause brain lesions and subsequent endocrine disorders when fed to the very young, and cause adverse reactions for all ages. These toxic products, plus others, are being poured into food, pharmaceuticals, dietary supplements, cosmetics, and infant formula — without restriction except for something called "good manufacturing practices." I find it fascinating — and a tribute to the power of the food and drug industries — that the cost of healthcare is ostensibly of great concern to our president and Congress, while the cost of pouring toxins into food isn't even considered.

As this is written, the FDA is on record as saying that consumers don't have the right to know what's in their food. At the same time, the FDA has approved the use of microparticulated chemical products in food. They're being advertised to industry as products to facilitate salt reduction, sugar replacement, MSG replacement, reduction of bitter taste in various food additives, and more. They've never been tested for safety, haven't been awarded GRAS status by the FDA, and will never be identified on the labels of foods in which they're used. The FDA has been asked by industry to allow it to classify these 100 percent chemicals as "natural flavors," instead of what they're known as now, "artificial flavors." Consumers will never know what they're ingesting, because these chemicals can be used in food, cosmetics, dietary supplements, and pharmaceuticals without disclosure.

But there's more to be considered than simple profits. There are the players. There are those who are orchestrating this pollution of our society, and those who enable it. Industry has built a system for ensuring its goals. It includes control of the regulators (both elected officials and regulatory agencies) and control of the media, which might otherwise expose what's being done to the public by industry. Industry has infiltrated every facet of our society: medical and regulatory. It's built a lobbying system that delivers funds to legislators, and rewards both legislators and agency staff with perks about which both exposés and novels have been written.

Today, human health and safety are being sacrificed for industry profits. While each industry reaps profits from its own contribution to pollution, be it pollution of the air, water, earth, or food, there's one industry — the pharmaceutical industry — that profits from it all.

Read the medical literature. There are a handful of researchers doing basic research. The rest are working on developing drugs to treat disease. Few, if any, work on preventing disease — unless prevention is cast in the form of a drug or vaccine (all with side effects) produced and sold by the pharmaceutical industry.

Today, those who promote use of vitamins, minerals, or other truly natural dietary supplements are being vilified. The FDA and/or USDA inspectors harass small organic farmers. Those who have treated diseases like cancer with far greater success than the mainstream medical community are hassled and intimidated. Anything that might cut into the profits of the pharmaceutical industry, be it simply providing healthy food to consumers, is routinely attacked, while toxic vaccines that have no track record of safety are being forced on our children.

Sometimes, when I lie in bed I think about these things, and wonder if the greedy are so greedy that they'll feed their own children and grandchildren food into which toxic chemicals have been poured. I think of dictators who are criticized for killing their own people. I wonder how different that is from the disabling and killing of Americans, done by those who pollute the air we're given to breathe and the food we're given to eat.

Yes, this book will be published, but the subject won't be closed. We know that MfG contains impurities. We know that MfG is an excitotoxic (brain damaging) amino acid. Thus, we know that the dose makes a difference. But we don't know how these two things — or if these two things — work together to do harm. Or if there's something more we know nothing about.

I often wonder if the truth about the toxicity of free glutamic acid will ever be acknowledged by our regulatory agencies. I also wonder if down the road it might occur to someone besides myself that the addition of excessive amounts of manufactured free glutamate (MfG) ingested in food might play a role in the increase of all kinds of disease and disability.

It's no secret that glutamate plays a role in neurodegenerative disease and more. But as this is written, the Glutes are calling the shots, and it's not politically correct to consider such a thing.

Notes

1. www.alzinfo.org/index.asp; and www.alzinfo.org/top-ten-alzheimers-signs-symptoms Accessed 7/5/2012. From a list of top 10 Alzheimer's Symptoms, a self-assessment tool developed by the Alzheimer's Association, taken from the web page of the Fisher Center for Alzheimer's Research Foundation.

2. Schwartz G. *In bad taste: the MSG syndrome.* Santa Fe: Health Press, 1988.

3. Filer LJ Jr., Garattini S, Kare MR, Reynolds WA, Wurtman RJ (Eds). *Glutamic acid: advance in biochemistry and physiology.* New York: Raven, 1979.

4. https://www.truthinlabeling.org/assets/seven_lines/Seven_Lines_Lines2.pdf Accessed 7/5/2021.

5. Olney JW. Excitotoxic amino acids: research applications and safety implications. In: Filer LJ Jr. et al. (Eds). *Glutamic acid: advance in biochemistry and physiology.* New York: Raven, 1979. pp 287-319.

6. Selected MSG-safety animal studies. www.truthinlabeling.org/IndustryAnimalSafetyStudies.htm

7. Selected MSG safety human studies.
www.truthinlabeling.org/IndustryHumanSafetyStudies.htm

8. Samuels A. The toxicity/safety of processed free glutamic acid (MSG): a study in suppression of information. *Account Res.* 1999;6:259-310. Also https://www.truthinlabeling.org/assets/manuscript2.pdf Accessed 6/24/2022.

9. The ABCs of flavor enhancement. *Prepared Foods.* August 1991. p 139.

10. Pszczola DE. "Friendly" labels: responding to consumer desires. *Food Technology.* May 1993. p 124.

11. Brown S. Annual ingredient update: a supplement to Dairy Field. June, 1993. p 8.

12. Rundlett KL, Armstrong DW. Evaluation of free D-glutamate in processed foods. *Chirality.* 1994; 6:277-282.

13. Deki M, Echizen A, Temma T. Minor components in monosodium glutamate. Bulletin of the Central Customs Laboratory. 1977; 17.

14. U.S. Patent #5,573,945. Mutant and method for producing L-glutamic acid by fermentation. Ajinomoto Co., Inc. (Tokyo, JP). November 12, 1996.
https://patents.google.com/patent/US5573945A/en
Accessed 6/24/2012.

15. Leung A, Foster S. *Encyclopedia of common natural ingredients used in food, drugs, and cosmetics.* New York: Wiley, 1996.

16. www.msgfacts.com/about_glutamate/msg_basics.aspx Accessed 7/6/2010.

17. www.msgfacts.com/about_glutamate/msg_basics.aspx

Accessed 7/6/2012.

18. Answers.com Food and Drug Administration.
https://www.fda.gov/food/food-additives-petitions/questions-and-ans
wers-monosodium-glutamate-msg
Accessed 7/5/2022.

19. *Los Angeles Times*, Staff and Wire Reports. California in Brief: San
Francisco: MSG Labeling Plan Causes Headaches. February 10, 1990.
articles.latimes.com/1990-02-10/news/mn-104_1_san-francisco.
Accessed 6/24/2012.

20. American Medical Association (AMA) Council on Scientific Affairs
(1991). (Resolution 187).

21. America Medical Association. Report of the Council on Scientific
Affairs: Food and Drug Administration regulations regarding the
inclusion of added L-glutamic acid content on food labels. Report: D
(A-92). 1992.
www.truthinlabeling.org/AMA.Policy_1992.pdf Accessed 7/8/2012.

22. Partial list of articles published by John W. Olney in 1982 and earlier.
www.truthinlabeling.org/pubmed_result_Pre1982.doc.htm
Accessed 6/25/2012.

23. *Food Chemical News*. "Reaction flavors" contain same components
as MSG, firm says. September 16, 1991. p 13.

24. Codex Alimentarius Commission, World Health Organization.
Joint FAO/WHO food standards programme, codex committee on food
additives and contaminants, Thirty-third Session, The Hague, March
12-16, 2001.
https://www.truthinlabeling.org/Codex_paper_on_chloroproponals.
pdf Accessed 10/30/2012.

25. *Food Chemical News*. May 31, 1993. p 16.

26. Ferguson GA. *Statistical analysis in psychology and education*. New York: McGraw-Hill, 1959.

27. Weinberg GH, Schumaker JA. Statistics: an intuitive approach. Belmont: Wadsworth, 1962.

28. McNemar Q. Psychological Statistics. New York: Wiley, 1949.

29. Ebert AG. Letter to Sue Ann Anderson, R.D., Ph.D., Senior Staff Scientist, FASEB. March 22, 1991. www.truthinlabeling.org/Ebert.AndersonLetter.pdf Accessed 6/25/2012.

30. Olney JW, Ho OL, Rhee V. Brain-damaging potential of protein hydrolysates. *N Engl J Med*. 1973; 289(8):391-5.

31. FDA Technical Information Specialist (HFS-728). Memorandum to Health Hazard Evaluation Board. Re: Summary of Adverse Reactions Attributed to Aspartame. June 26, 1997. https://truthinlabeling.org/assets/arms_aspartame.pdf

32. Ebert AG. Presentation: Evaluation of amino acids and related products. FASEB/LSRO, February 4, 1991. (Ace-Federal Reporters, Inc. 800-336-6646)

33. Crichton M. *Rising sun*. New York: Ballantine, 2008.

34. Federation of American Societies for Experimental Biology, Life Sciences Research Office Report: Health aspects of dietary trans fatty acids. Prepared for Center for Food Safety and Applied Nutrition, Food and Drug Administration. Bethesda, MD, 1985.

35. International Food Information Council. MSG Committee/MSG Coalition. (1991). Communications Plan, July-December 1991 (As revised at 7/22/91 meeting).

36. Burros M. Corporate support to dietitians group is called unhealthy.

New York Times. November 15, 1995. p B1.

37. Chinese restaurant syndrome: Putting a mysterious ailment into perspective. *Mayo Clinic Nutrition Letter.* January, 1990.

38. University of California at Berkeley Wellness Letter. University of California at Berkeley School of Public Health. October, 1989.

39. University of California at Berkeley Wellness Letter. University of California at Berkeley School of Public Health. June 1996. p 2.

40. Wood J. Are you sensitive to 'harmless' MSG? *Modern Maturity.* August- September 1991, pp 34:74.

41. Samuels A. MSG: a review of the literature and critique of industry sponsored research. (unpublished) 1991. www.truthinlabeling.org/REV.html Accessed 7/8/2012.

42. Filer LJ Jr, Stegink LD. A report of the proceedings of an MSG workshop held August 1991. *Crit Rev Food Sci Nutr.* 1994; 34(2):159-74.

43. Fernstrom JD, Garattini S, (Eds). International symposium on glutamate. *J Nutr.* 2000; 130:4S. pp 891S-1079S.

44. Ingersol B. TV jitters: food industry awaits with queasy stomach a '60 minutes' show. *Wall Street Journal.* October 17, 1991. p 1

45. Commonwealth of Pennsylvania Plaintiff v Pepperidge Farm, Incorporated Defendant. Civil Action Equity No 257 M.D. 1991. https://www.truthinlabeling.org/Labeling-PepperidgeFarm_ AttorneysGeneral.pdf

46. Commonwealth of Pennsylvania Plaintiff v. Matlaw's Food Products, Inc., Respondents, Civil Action Equity No. 231 M.D. 1991.

47. Commonwealth of Pennsylvania Plaintiff v. S&B International

Corporation, Defendant. Civil Action Equity No. 358 MD 1992.
www.truthinlabeling.org/Labeling-S&B_AttorneysGeneral.pdf

48. People of the State of California v. Union Inc., a California
Corporation doing business as Union Foods. Civil Action: CIV 111845.
Suit filed in Ventura County Superior Court, 1990.
www.truthinlabeling.org\Labeling-VenturaCounty.pdf

49. Kelley D. Company pays $13,000 for false claim on MSG. *Los Angeles
Times*. July 7, 1990.

50. FDA. FDA Regulatory Letter to Fantastic Foods, Inc., Novato, CA.
April 10, 1990.
www.truthinlabeling.org\Labeling-FDA.FantasticFoods.pdf

51. *Food Chemical News*. May 31, 1993. p 16.

52. Lin LJ. Presentation: Regulatory status of maillard reactions flavors,
Washington DC: Division of Food and Color Additives, Center for
Food Safety and Applied Nutrition, Food and Drug Administration.
Paper presented at a meeting of the American Chemical Society, August
24, 1992.

53. Pommer K. New Proteoloytic enzymes for the production of savory
ingredients. *Cereal Foods World*. 1995; 40(10):745-748.

54. *Food Chemical News*, Dec 2, 1996. pp 24-25.

55. National Toxicology Program (NTP) of the National Institute of
Environmental Health Sciences (NIEHS) at the National Institutes of
Health (NIH). 1,3-Dichloro-2-propanol [CAS No. 96-23-1] Review of
Toxicological Literature. January, 2005
www.truthinlabeling.org/NIH_dichloropropanol_2005.pdf
Accessed 7/8/2012.

56. Codex Alimentarius Commission Position Paper on
Chloropropanols. The Hague, The Netherlands, March 12-16, 2001.

www.truthinlabeling.org/Codex_paper_on_chloroproponals.pdf
Accessed 7/8/2012.

57. *Food Chemical News.* FDA reviewing MSG as possible excitotoxin, Hattan says. August 6, 1990. p 12.

58. Federation of American Societies for Experimental Biology (FASEB). Safety of amino acids used as dietary supplements. Bethesda, MD: Life Sciences Research Office, FASEB. July 1992.

59. Ebert A. Acknowledgment of invitation: FDA Food Advisory Committee. September 10, 1992.

60. McNutt K. Bio.
www.mcnuttwebsite.com/ABMcNuttBio.html Accessed 7/8/2012.

61. Hattan DG. Letter to Mr. Jack Samuels and Dr. Adrienne Samuels. December 1, 1993.

62. Maddox CC. Letter to Adrienne Samuels. January 31, 1995.

63. US Department of Health and Human Services. Office of Research Integrity. ori.hhs.gov/about-ori Accessed 7/8/2012.

64. FDA. Contract between the FDA and the Life Sciences Research office of the Federation of American Societies for Experimental Biology (LSRO/FASEB), signed on February 1, 1995, FDA Contract 223-92-2185.

65. Life Sciences research Office Federation of American Societies for Experimental Biology. Tentative report: Adequacy of existing scientific information on possible adverse reactions to monosodium glutamate. February, 1993.

66. Life Sciences research Office Federation of American Societies for Experimental Biology. Tentative report: Adequacy of existing scientific information on possible adverse reactions to monosodium glutamate. II.

Scope of the Tentative Report. February, 1993. pp 3-5.

67. Nemeroff CB. Monosodium glutamate-induced neurotoxicity: review of the literature and call for further research. In: *Nutrition & Behavior* Miller SA, (Ed.) Philadelphia: The Franklin Institute Press, 1981.

68. Olney JW. Prepared statement pertaining to adverse reactions to monosodium glutamate (MSG). Presented at a public meeting conducted by the Federation of American Societies for Experimental Biology (FASEB), Bethesda, MD. April, 1993. In: Samuels A. The toxicity/safety of processed free glutamic acid (MSG): a study in suppression of information. Appendix B. Account Res. 1999; 6:259-310. FDA Docket 92N-0391 (TS7). www.truthinlabeling.org/l-manuscript.html Accessed 6/24/2012. Also, www.truthinlabeling.org/l-append.html Accessed 10/30/2012

69. Henneberry RC. Presentation: Analysis of adverse reactions to monosodium glutamate (MSG). FDA Docket No. 92N-0391. Presentation made before FASEB, Bethesda, MD, April 7, 1993.

70. Frieder B, Grimm VE. Prenatal monosodium glutamate (MSG) treatment given through the mother's diet causes behavioral deficits in rat offspring. *Intern J Neurosci.* 1984; 23:117-126.

71. Frieder B, Grimm VE. Prenatal monosodium glutamate. *Neurochem.* 1987; 48:1359-1365.

72. Tarasoff L, Kelly MF. Monosodium L glutamate: a double blind study and review. *Food Chem Toxic.* 1993; 31:1019 35.

73. Samuels A. Monosodium L-glutamate: a double-blind study and review. Letter to the editor. *Food and Chemical Toxicology.* 1995; 33:69-78.

74. Ebert AG. Letter to Fred Shank, Director, Center for food Safety and Applied Nutrition, FDA from the International Glutamate Technical

Committee. January 2, 1991.

75. Ho T. Letter to Dr. A. Samuels. June 1, 1994.

76. Blaylock RL. *Excitotoxins: the taste that kills*. Santa Fe: Health Press, 1994

77. Pratt S. Flavor-enhancing Msg is everywhere, but is it harmless or an 'excitotoxin'? *Chicago Tribune*, July 28, 1994. articles.chicagotribune.com/1994-07-28/entertainment/9407280144_1_glutamates-msg-brain-barrier Accessed 7/9/2012.

78. Pratt S. '60 Minutes' report on MSG triggers more debate. *Chicago Tribune*, November 7, 1991. articles.chicagotribune.com/1991-11-07/entertainment/9104100250_1_free-glutamate-labeling-flavor- enhancer Accessed 7/9/2012.

79. Eng M, Deardorff J. Navigating the MSG maze. *Chicago Tribune*, November 24, 2008. articles.chicagotribune.com/2008-11-24/news/0811230241_1_msg-glutamates-soups Accessed 7/9/2012.

80. Burton Goldberg Group. Alternative medicine: the definitive guide. Puyallup, WA: *Future Medicine Pub.*, 1993.

81. On the subject of manufactured vs natural glutamic acid. www.truthinlabeling.org/manufac.html Accessed 7/2/2012.

82. Healing Edge Sciences, Inc. www.healingedge.net/store/article_supplement_facts.html Accessed 7/9/2012.

83. US Pharmacopeial Convention. Food Chemicals Codex. www.usp.org/support-home/frequently-asked-questions/food-chemicals-codex-fcc Accessed 7/9/2012

84. International Glutamate Technical Committee. Letter from Yoshihisa Sugita to Daniel J. Raiten, Life Sciences Research Office, Federation of American Societies for Experimental Biology. January 26, 1994.

85. Samuels A. Evidence of MSG-induced brain damage and endocrine disorders: the animal studies. Compiled May, 2009. www.truthinlabeling.org/Proof_BrainLesions_CNS.htm Accessed 7/9/2012.

86. Olney JW. Personal communication.

87. International Symposium on Glutamate. Fernstrom JD, Garattini S, (Eds). J Nutr. 2000; 130: 891S. jn.nutrition.org/content/130/4/891.full.pdf Accessed 7/2/2012.

88. Truth in Labeling Campaign, et al., Plaintiffs, v. Donna Shalala, et al., Defendants. No. 4:95CV1633 TCM.

89. Monsanto. Aspartame/Nutrasweet monsanto.com/newsviews/Pages/aspartame-nutrasweet.aspx Accessed 7/2/2012.

90. Chemical Online. JW Childs Acquires Monsanto's NutraSweet Sweetener Business, March 28, 2000. www.chemicalonline.com/doc.mvc/JW-Childs-Acquires-Monsantos-NutraSweet-Sweet-0001 Accessed 7/2/2012.

91. Olney JW. Prepared statement pertaining to adverse reactions to monosodium glutamate (MSG). Presented at a public meeting conducted by the Federation of American Societies for Experimental Biology (FASEB), Bethesda, MD. April, 1993. In: Samuels A. The toxicity/safety of processed free glutamic acid (MSG): a study in suppression of information. Appendix B. Account Res. 1999; 6:259-310. FDA Docket 92N-0391 (TS7). www.truthinlabeling.org/assets/manuscript2.pdf Accessed 6/24/2012. Also, www.truthinlabeling.org/l-append.html Accessed 10/30/2012.

92. Simon RA, Stevenson DD, Scripps Clinic and Research Foundation, La Jolla, California. Letter to David A. Kessler, M.D. Commissioner of Food and Drug Administration. August 30, 1995.

93. Federation of American Societies for Experimental Biology (FASEB). Analysis of adverse reactions to monosodium glutamate (MSG). Bethesda, MD: Life Sciences Research Office, FASEB, 1995.

94. Procardia side effects. Drugs.com www.drugs.com/sfx/procardia-side-effects.html Accessed 7/2/2012.

95. Nambudripad's Allergy Elimination Techniques www.naet. com/ Accessed 7/2/2012.

96. Nambudripad DS. *Say goodbye to illness*. Buena Park, CA: Delta, 1993.

97. International Glutamate Technical Committee (IGTC). *The Encyclopedia of Associations*, 26th Edition, 1992.

98. International Glutamate Technical Committee (IGTC). *National Trade and Professional Associations of the United States*, 1994 Edition, 1994.

99. Glutamate Association U.S. *The Encyclopedia of Associations*, 24th Edition, 1990.

100. Food Technology. Chicago: Institute of Food Technologists. September, 1993. p 34.

101. Taylor SL. Possible adverse reactions to hydrolyzed vegetable protein. Paper submitted to the Federation of American Societies for Experimental Biology review panel. April, 1993.

102. Taylor SL. Presentation: Food Allergies and Sensitivities. SciTalk, National Health Museum.

www.accessexcellence.org/LC/ST/st14presbio.php
Accessed 7/2/2012

103. The food allergy and anaphylaxis network. Medical advisory board.
www.foodallergy.org/page/medical-advisory-board
Accessed 10/30/2012/

104. Macrae R, Robinson RK, Sadler MJ, (Eds.) *Encyclopedia of Food Science Food Technology and Nutrition*. London: Academic Press, 1993.

105. Taylor SL. Letter to FDA Dockets Management Branch. July 26, 1991.

106. Taylor SL, Hefle SL. Letter to FDA Dockets Management Branch Re: Food Labeling Declaration of Free Glutamate in Food (Docket 96N-0244). March 7, 1997.

107. Kenney RA, Tidball CS. Human susceptibility to oral monosodium L-glutamate. *A J Clin Nutr.* 1972; 25:140-146.

108. Auer RN. Excitotoxic mechanisms, and age-related susceptibility to brain damage in ischemia, hypoglycemia and toxic mussel poisoning. *Neuro Toxicology.* 1991; 12:541-546.

109. Kenney RA. Placebo-controlled studies of human reaction to oral monosodium L-glutamate. In: Filer LJ Jr, Garattini S, Kare MR, Reynolds WA, Wurtman RJ, (Eds). *Glutamic acid: advances in biochemistry and physiology*. New York: Raven, 1979.

110. Auer RN. Expert Report of Roland N. Auer, M.D., Ph.D., F.R.C.P.C. Statement made on behalf of the U.S. Department of Health and Human Services, Office of the General Counsel, Food and Drug Division, Rockville, MD 20857, September 30, 1996.

111. Ebert AG. Curriculum vitae.

112. Ebert AG. Letters to the Editor: Evidence That MSG Does Not

Induce Obesity. Obesity. 2009; 17(4):629–630.
www.nature.com/oby/journal/v17/n4/full/oby2008631a.html
Accessed 3/16/2012.

113. FDA. Memorandum of Conference. Center for Food Safety and Applied Nutrition, FDA. Subject: the research of R.S. Geha (Harvard Medical School), A. Saxon (UCLA Medical School), R. Patterson (Northwestern University Medical School), and the IGTC. October 23, 1992.

114. Ajinomoto. About us.
ajinomoto.com/about/corporateguidance/directors/index.html

115. United States Patent Office.
https://patents.google.com/patent/US3387028

116. YouTube.
www.youtube.com/watch?v=WM6kV6OYY_Y Accessed 3/16/2012.

117. United States Pharmacopeial Convention (USP).
www.usp. org/aboutUSP/ Accessed 6/29/2010.

118. Ebert AG. Letter to David A. Kessler, Commissioner of Food and Drugs Department of Health & Human Services Food and Drug Administration. September 9, 1992.

119. Metcalfe DD, Sampson HA, Simon RA, (Eds). Food Allergy: Adverse Reactions to Foods and Food Additives. Oxford: Blackwell, 1991.

120. Allen D. Personal communication. August 20, 1990.

121. Simon RA, Stevenson DD, Scripps Clinic and Research Foundation, La Jolla, California. Letter to David A. Kessler, M.D. Commissioner of Food and Drug Administration. August 30, 1995.

122. Stevenson DD, Simon RA, Woessner KM. The role of

monosodium L-glutamate (MSG) in asthma: does it exist? Poster
presentation #1670. AAAAI/AAI/CIS joint meeting. American
Academy of Allergy Asthma & Immonology. San Francisco, CA.
February 25, 1997.

123. Schwartz K. NoMSG Messenger (Newsletter of the National
Organization Mobilized to Stop Glutamate). Summer, 1996.

124. Samuels A. Letter to Dr. Ronald Simon. May 24, 1997.

125. Simon R. Letter to Adrienne Samuels, Ph.D. May 28, 1997.

126. Olney JW, Price MT. Neuroendocrine interactions of excitatory
and inhibitory amino acids. *Brain Research Bulletin.* 1980; 5(Suppl
2):361- 368.

127. Olney JW, Price MT. Excitotoxic amino acids as neuroendocrine
probes. In: *Kainic Acid a Tool in Neurobiology.* McGeer, EG, et al., (Eds).
New York: Raven Press, 1978.

128. Morselli P, Garattini S. Monosodium-glutamate and the Chinese
restaurant syndrome. *Nature.* 1970; 227:611-612.

129. Bazzano G, D'Elia JA, Olson RE. Monosodium glutamate: feeding
of large amounts in man and gerbils. *Science.* 1970; 169:1208-1209.

130. FDA Advanced Notice of Proposed Rulemaking. Federal Register,
September 12, 1996, pp 48102-48110.

131. Olney JW. Glutamate-induced neuronal necrosis in the infant
mouse hypothalamus. *J Neuropathol Exp Neurol.* 1971; 30:75-90.

132. Burde RM, Schainker B, Kayes J. Acute effect of oral and
subcutaneous administration of monosodium glutamate on the arcuate
nucleus of the hypothalamus in mice and rats. *Nature* (Lond). 1971;
233:58-60.

133. Olney JW, Sharpe LG, Feigin RD. Glutamate-induced brain damage in infant primates. *J Neuropathol Exp Neurol*. 1972; 31:464-488.

134. Burde RM, Schainker, B, Kayes J. Monosodium glutamate: necrosis of hypothalamic neurons in infant rats and mice following either oral or subcutaneous administration. *J Neuropathol Exp Neurol*. 1972; 31:181.

135. Olney JW, Ho OL. Brain damage in infant mice following oral intake of glutamate, aspartate or cystine. *Nature* (Lond). 1970; 227:609-611.

136. Lemkey-Johnston N, Reynolds WA. Incidence and extent of brain lesions in mice following ingestion of monosodium glutamate (MSG). *Anat Rec*. 1972; 172:354.

137. Takasaki, Y. Protective effect of mono- and disaccharides on glutamate- induced brain damage in mice. *Toxicol Lett*. 1979; 4:205-210.

138. Takasaki, Y. Protective effect of arginine, leucine, and preinjection of insulin on glutamate neurotoxicity in mice. *Toxicol Lett*. 1980; 5:39-44.

139. Lemkey-Johnston N. Reynolds WA. Nature and extent of brain lesions in mice related to ingestion of monosodium glutamate: a light and electron microscope study. *J Neuropath Exp Neurol*. 1974; 33:74-97.

140 Olney JW. Brain lesions, obesity, and other disturbances in mice treated with monosodium glutamate. *Science*. 1969; 164:719-721.

141 Filer LJ, Stegink L.D. Safety of hydrolysates in parenteral nutrition. *N Engl J Med*. 1973; 289:426-427.

142 Olney JW, Ho OL, Rhee V, DeGubareff T. Neurotoxic effects of glutamate. *New Engl J Med*. 1973; 289:1374-1375.

143. Olney JW, Ho OL, Rhee V. Cytotoxic effects of acidic and sulphur containing amino acids on the infant mouse central nervous system. *Exp Brain Res.* 1971; 14(1):61-76.

144. Reynolds WA, Lemkey-Johnston N, Filer LJ Jr., Pitkin RM. Monosodium Glutamate: absence of hypothalamic lesions after ingestion by newborn primates. *J Neuropath Exp Neurol.* 1972; 31:181-182. (Abstract)

145. Olney JW, Sharpe LG, Feigin RD. Glutamate-induced brain damage in infant primates. *J Neuropathol Exp Neurol.* 1972; 31:464-488.

146. Burde RM, Schainker B, Kayes J. Acute effect of oral and subcutaneous administration of monosodium glutamate on the arcuate nucleus of the hypothalamus in mice and rats. *Nature.* 1971; 233(5314):58-60.

147. Mears JA, Assistant to the President, University of Iowa. Iowa City, Iowa. Letter to Adrienne Samuels. August 29, 1991. www.truthinlabeling.org/Filer_re.Mead-Johnson_Professor_ FromU.of.Iowa.pdf

148. Filer LJ. Public Forum: analysis of adverse reactions to monosodium glutamate. Paper presented at open meeting of the Federation of American Societies for Experimental Biology, April 1993.

149. National Academy of Sciences National Research Council. Safety and suitability of monosodium glutamate for use in baby foods. July, 1970.

150. Gillette R. Academy food committees: new criticism of industry ties. *Science.* 1972; 177:1172-1175.

151. Geha R, Beiser A, Ren C, Patterson R, Greenberger P, Grammer LC, Ditto AM, Harris KE, Shaughnessy MA, Yarnold P, Corren J, Saxon A. Multicenter multiphase double blind placebo controlled study to evaluate alleged reactions to monosodium glutamate (MSG). *J Allergy Clin Immunol Abstracts.* 1998; 101:S243 (Abstract 106).

152. Geha RS, Beiser A, Ren C, Patterson R, Greenberger PA, Grammer LC, Ditto AM, Harris KE, Shaughnessy MA, Yarnold PR, Corren J, Saxon A. Multicenter, double-blind, placebo-controlled, multiple-challenge evaluation of reported reactions to monosodium glutamate. *J Allergy Clin Immunol.* 2000 Nov; 106(5):973-80.

153. Geha RS, Beiser A, Ren C, Patterson R, Greenberger PA, Grammer LC, Ditto AM, Harris KE, Shaughnessy MA, Yarnold PR, Corren J, Saxon A. Review of alleged reaction to monosodium glutamate and outcome of a multicenter double-blind placebo-controlled study. *J Nutr.* 2000 Apr; 130(4S Suppl):1058S-62S.

154. Goldschmiedt M, Redfern JS, Feldman M. Food coloring and monosodium glutamate: effects on the cephalic phase of gastric acid secretion and gastrin release in humans. *Am J Clin Nutr.* 1990; 51:794-797.

155. Ebert AG. Letter to Walter H. Glinsmann, M.D., Associate Director of Clinical Nutrition, Division of Nutrition, FDA. Subject: the research of Donald Kirby, M.D., Medical College of Virginia. July 13, 1990.

156. Wolke RL. Food 101: the mystery of MSG. *Washington Post.* June 17, 1998. pp E1-E2.

157. FDA. Summary of adverse reactions attributed to MSG. www.truthinlabeling.org/FDA_ARMS_MSG.1997.pdf Accessed 8/28/2012.

158. Pommer K. (Novo Nordisk BioChem Inc., Franklinton, NC) *Cereal Foods World.* October, 1995; 40(10):745.

159. *Food Chemical News.* August 6, 1990. pp 10-12.

160. Daniels DH, Joe F, Diachenko GW. Determination of free glutamic acid in a variety of foods by high-performance liquid chromatography. *Food Additives and Contaminants.* 1995; 12:21-29.

161. Shepherd P. (Elsevier Science) Letter to Dr. Adrienne Samuels. February 9, 1995.

162. Ebert AG. Letter to Walter H. Glinsmann, M.D., Associate Director of Clinical Nutrition, Division of Nutrition, FDA. Subject: the research of Donald Kirby, M.D., Medical College of Virginia. July 13, 1990.

163. Burros M. Corporate support to dietitians group is called unhealthy. *New York Times.* November 15, 1995.

164. ADA Courier. An update for member of the American Dietetic Association. Volume 34, Number 11, November/December 1995.

165. American College of Allergy and Immunology. News release. 1991.

166. American College of Allergy, Asthma and Immunology (ACAAI). Position Statement on Monosodium Glutamate. ACAAI: Arlington Heights, Illinois. 1991.

167. American College of Allergy, Asthma and Immunology (ACAAI). Position Statement on Monosodium Glutamate. ACAAI: Arlington Heights, Illinois. 1991.

168. Institute of Food Technologists Expert Panel on Food Safety and Nutrition. Monosodium Glutamate, A Scientific Status Summary. Chicago: Institute of Food Technologists, 1980.

169. Mayo Clinic Nutrition Letter. Chinese restaurant syndrome. *Mayo Clinic Nutrition Letter.* January 1990.

170. Schmitz A. MSG: a cause for alarmists. *In Health.* November/ December 1990. pp 20-23.

171. McNutt K. Nutrition, Communications and the Information

Explosion. Presentation before the Society for Nutrition Education Metro-DC Affiliate. May 22, 1991.

172. Taliaferro PJ. Monosodium glutamate and the Chinese restaurant syndrome: a review of food additive safety. *J Environmental Health.* 1995; 57:8-12.

173. Tufts University Diet and Nutrition Letter. February 1992. pp 4-6.

174. Wood J. Are you sensitive to 'harmless' MSG? *Modern Maturity.* August- September 1991. pp 34-74.

175. University of California at Berkeley Wellness Letter. University of California at Berkeley School of Public Health. October, 1989.

176. University of California at Berkeley Wellness Letter. University of California at Berkeley School of Public Health. June 1996. p. 2.

177. International Food Information Council [IFIC]. MSG Committee/ MSG Coalition, Communications Plan, July-December, 1991 (As revised at 7/22/91 meeting).

178. International Food Information Council (1996). *The Encyclopedia of Associations,* 31st Edition.

179. Umami information center. Sweet, sour, salty, bitter and UMAMI. www.umamiinfo.com/images/stories/publications/sw_so_sa_bi_and_ umami_sample.pdf Accessed 10/30/2012.

180. Food Insight. Washington, DC: International Food Information Council (IFIC) Foundation. May/June 1994.

181. American Marketing Association. www.marketingpower.com/AboutAMA/Pages/DefinitionofMarketin g.aspx Accessed 3/16/2012.

182. The Free Dictionary.

legaldictionary.thefreedictionary.com/Lobbying Accessed 3/16/2012.

183. Allen DH, Delohery MB, Baker G. Monosodium L-glutamate-induced asthma. *J allergy clin immunol.* 1987; 80(4):530-537.

184. Select Committee on GRAS Substances. SCOGS-37a. Evaluation of the health aspects of certain glutamates as food ingredients. Prepared for the Food and Drug Administration by the Life Sciences Research Office, Federation of American Societies for Experimental Biology under contract No. FDA 223-75-2004. Available from Special Publications Office, FASEB, Bethesda, MD, 1978.

185. Select Committee on GRAS Substances. SCOGS-37a-supplement. Evaluation of the health aspects of certain glutamates as food ingredients. Prepared for the Food and Drug Administration by the Life Sciences Research Office, Federation of American Societies for Experimental Biology under contract No. FDA 223-75-2004. Available from Special Publications Office, FASEB, Bethesda, MD, 1980.

186. Federal Register: 61 FR 48102. 21 CFR part 101; FDA Docket No. 96N-0244, Document Number: 96-23159. Health and Human Services Department; Food Labeling; Declaration of Free Glutamate in Food: A Proposed Rule; 9/12/1996. http://federalregister.gov/a/96-23159 Accessed 3/16/2012.

187. Hahn MJ, Executive Director, The Glutamate Association. Letter to Docket 02N-0434. www.fda.gov/ohrms/DOCKETS/dailys/03/jul03/072803/02N-0434_emc-000005-01.PDF Accessed 3/16/2012

188. FDA. Summary of adverse reactions attributed to aspartame. www.truthinlabeling.org/FDA_ARMS_Asp.1997.pdf   Accessed 8/28/2012.

189. Lin LJ. Letter to Adrienne Samuels re: solicitation of adverse reactions reports. September 26, 1995.

190. Ebert AG. Letter to Walter H. Glinsmann, M.D. Subject: research of Donald Kirby, M.D. Medical College of Virginia, July 13, 1990.

191. Ebert AG. Letter to Fred R. Shank, Ph.D. Director, CFSAN, FDA. Subject: request for a scientific review session on MSG with FDA scientists. January 2, 1991.

192. FDA. Memorandum of Conference. Center for Food Safety and Applied Nutrition, FDA. Subject: the research of R.S. Geha (Harvard Medical School), A. Saxon (UCLA Medical School), R. Patterson (Northwestern University Medical School), and the IGTC. October 23, 1992.

193. Smolinske SC. *Handbook of food, drug, and cosmetic excipients.* Boca Raton: CRC Press, 1992.

194. National Institutes of Health. The glutamate cascade: common pathways of central nervous system disease states. Bethesda, Maryland. May 3-5, 1998 conference.
https://archives.drugabuse.gov/es/meetings/1998/05/glutamate-cascade
-common-pathways-central-nervous-system-disease-states

195. Brown Harriet. How Obesity Became a Disease - And, as a consequence, how weight loss became an industry. *The Atlantic.* March 24, 2015.

196. Brown, Harriet. *Body of Truth.* Boston, Da Capo Press, 2015.

Appendix

Industry's FDA

The FDA's cooperation with Ajinomoto to promote the use of monosodium glutamate (MSG) was first evidenced in 1969 during testimony given before the Senate Select Committee on Nutrition and Health on the safety of MSG by then FDA Commissioner Herbert Ley. Commissioner Ley testified to four studies that allegedly demonstrated the safety of MSG. It was later confirmed that two of those studies had not been completed, and the others didn't exist.

Since that time FDA/industry cooperation has included:

- **Telling blatant lies** about the safety of MSG, lies originating with the glutamate industry and repeated by the FDA.

- **Dispensing complimentary information** about MSG while withholding information that might be considered negative.

- **Officially approving study protocols** for MSG-is-safe studies that used placebos known to cause the same reactions as those caused by MSG test material.

- **Allowing glutamate-industry propaganda** to be displayed on the FDA webpage.

- **Refusing to collect reports** of reactions to MSG "because we know that no one reacts to MSG."

- **Withholding key information** from dietitians, nutritionists, consumers, and the medical community.

Information withheld from dietitians, nutritionists, consumers, and the medical community includes:

- The glutamate in MSG, and therefore MSG itself, is excitotoxic – brain damaging.

- There is a second excitotoxic amino acid used in food. It's the aspartic acid component of "sugar-free" or "low calorie" sweeteners with names such as aspartame, Equal, NutraSweet and AminoSweet.

- When used in pharmaceuticals, glutamic acid is regulated as a drug. When used in food, glutamate is regulated as a food.

- When use in pharmaceuticals, the many and varied reactions following use of glutamic acid are called side effects.

- When used in food, the many and varied reactions following ingestion of glutamate-containing MSG are not acknowledged as side effects of glutamic acid, although that's exactly what they are.

- Adverse reactions known to be caused by excitotoxic manufactured free glutamate (MfG) are many and varied, ranging from simple skin rash to anaphylactic shock.

- When used as a discrete ingredient in processed food, excitotoxic manufactured free glutamate (MfG) will be labeled glutamic acid, L-glutamic acid, L-glutamate, glutamate or E620.

- MfG is also found as a constituent of ingredients that contain glutamate that has been freed from protein during fermentation or other forms of processing. These include, but are not limited to, anything "hydrolyzed," "autolyzed" or "enzyme-modified." The list of ingredients known at this time to contain MfG can be found at https://www.truthinlabeling.org/names.html

- Manufactured free glutamic acid (MfG) is always accompanied by unwanted by-products of manufacture, referred to as impurities. There are impurities associated with the L-glutamate in monosodium glutamate (since monosodium glutamate is manufactured), but there are no similar impurities in the intact protein found in the human body.

- The popular method for producing monosodium glutamate today calls for feeding carefully selected genetically modified bacteria on a diet that will enable the bacteria to secrete glutamic acid through their cell walls. There have been a variety of such methods used since 1957– many, if not all of which, are patented.

- Monosodium glutamate exerts its influence on receptors in the central nervous system and glutamate receptors in many peripheral tissues, including lungs, heart, and skin. It can excite — and over-excite — receptors in the brain and central nervous system, and also excite and over-excite receptor cells in the heart, kidney, lungs, ovary, testis, liver, endocrine tissues, bone, and immune system, for example.

- There may be some small amount of free glutamic acid in unprocessed, unadulterated, food, but if so, it will not cause brain damage or adverse reactions. It is conceivable, but has not been demonstrated, that the impurities in manufactured free glutamate contribute to MSG-induced brain damage and adverse reactions. In this area, as in many others, research is sorely needed.

- The studies of the 1970s demonstrating that glutamic acid causes brain lesions were so well done and so often replicated that by the 1980's glutamic acid was being used by researchers as a tool to selectively kill brain cells. It is still used for that purpose in the laboratory.

- Monosodium glutamate stimulates glutamate receptors in the mouth and on the tongue (often referred to as taste buds by the glutamate industry). That results in producing perception of more taste in the food being eaten than would otherwise be perceived.

It is (or was), an FDA rule to investigate the reports of life-threatening reactions to FDA-regulated substances, however, such investigations have not been routinely executed.

In addition, on at least two separate occasions for which we have documentation, medical records of life-threatening reactions to MSG were altered/falsified.

The FDA has pretended to be concerned with public health, but has refused to require that processed free glutamic acid in processed foods, infant formula, enteral care products, protein powders, cosmetics, pharmaceuticals, and dietary supplements be labeled, so consumers could avoid it if they chose to do so.

In 1989, Jack Samuels and George Schwartz met with ranking members of the FDA to discuss what Samuels and Schwartz referred to as the hazards of consuming monosodium glutamate. Schwartz did all of the talking, and Samuels took minutes of the meeting. When the requested official FDA minutes of the meeting were received by Schwartz and Samuels, they found the only similarity between their copy and the FDA's was the names of the people who had attended.

A 50-YEAR HISTORY OF FDA/
GLUTAMATE-INDUSTRY COOPERATION

The FDA makes and enforces food labeling laws, and it is the FDA that determines whether or not MSG, or any other chemical, will be approved for use in food. The FDA has been cooperating with Ajinomoto Company, Inc., members of its International Glutamate Technical Committee (IGTC) and The Glutamate Association, and with the International Hydrolyzed Protein Council since at least 1968. The bottom line of that cooperative effort as it pertains to regulation of MSG is to prevent full and clear disclosure of MSG in processed food, or any other product or drug where it may be added.

Glutamate industry involvement in FDA matters is rarely obvious. That's what makes it so effective in preventing meaningful labeling of

MSG. FDA/industry cooperation can be traced back to 1958, when "monosodium glutamate" was first deemed "safe" by the FDA.

MSG could be deemed to be safe because prior to the 1958 implementation of the Food Additives Amendment to the Federal Food, Drug, and Cosmetic Act, there had been no record of adverse reactions to monosodium glutamate. But what was known as MSG prior to 1958 was replaced in 1957 by **a different product** also **called** MSG that was made using genetically modified bacteria. The FDA took no notice of the change.

It was not until 1968 that the first report of adverse reactions to monosodium glutamate was published in *The New England Journal of Medicine*, and not until 1969 that the first evidence that monosodium glutamate caused brain lesions and endocrine disorders in laboratory animals was published in *Science*.

The FDA has built and then reinforced its case for the "safety" of MSG on misleading and deceptive studies sponsored by the glutamate industry. FDA regulations require that those who manufacture food additives must provide evidence demonstrating that they are "safe." The glutamate industry has, indeed, presented evidence, but they have falsified data — not by changing test scores or research results, but by rigging the procedures used in conducting their studies so that only after careful scrutiny could one discern that their studies were flawed to the point of being fraudulent. Glutamate industry studies are generally methodologically inadequate, statistically unsound, and/or irrelevant to the safety/toxicity of MSG. Researchers have gone so far as to use aspartame and/or MSG in placebos to cause subjects to respond to placebos just as they would respond to monosodium glutamate test material. In addition, industry's researchers have been known to draw conclusions that did not follow from the results of their studies.

Over the course of the last 50 years, the FDA has summarily dismissed much of the research that clearly demonstrates that MSG places humans at risk, not by countering it, but simply ignoring it. Reports of adverse reactions to MSG grudgingly collected by its own Adverse Reactions Monitoring System have been dismissed because "they could have been caused by something else."

The FDA has suppressed results of studies that might suggest that use of MSG places humans at risk. The FDA suppressed results of its own study that suggested that use of free glutamic acid in supplements is unsafe. In a July 1992, report to the FDA, the Federation of American Societies for Experimental Biology (FASEB) had concluded, in part, that:

> "...it is prudent to avoid the use of dietary supplements of L-glutamic acid by pregnant women, infants, and children.... and...by women of childbearing age and individuals with affective disorders."

MSG is called L-glutamic acid when used in supplements. Mention has not been made of those recommendations – not to the medical community or anywhere else.

Books have been written detailing FDA corruption. The following are examples:

Eating May Be Hazardous To Your Health — The Case Against Food Additives, by Jacqueline Verrett and Jean Carper

Health at Gunpoint: The FDA's Silent War Against Health Freedom (Paperback), by James Gormley

The Rise Of Tyranny (Paperback), by Jonathan W. Emord

Codex Alimentarius Global Food Imperialism by Scott Tips

Inside the FDA: The Business and Politics Behind the Drugs We Take and the Food We Eat (Hardcover), by Fran Hawthorne

Stolen Harvest: The Hijacking of the Global Food Supply (Paperback), by Vandana Shiva

The Truth about the Drug Companies: How They Deceive Us and What to Do about It (Paperback), by Marcia Angell

The FDA has refused to recall foods advertised as "No MSG," "No Added MSG," or "No MSG Added" even though those foods contain ingredients that are sources of free glutamic acid such as hydrolyzed protein, and are, therefore, in direct violation of Section 403(a)(1) of the Federal Food, Drug, and Cosmetic Act.

FDA practice has included distributing unsolicited copies of an FDA Medical Bulletin that assures physicians that MSG is safe. Similar material has been distributed to food service people.

FDA practice has included reviewing the subject of monosodium glutamate safety favorably in "The FDA Consumer," "Talk Papers," "Backgrounders," "FDA Consumer MEMO's," pamphlets such as "Food Additives" — (FDA done in Cooperation with IFIC), and sending out packets labeled "Consumer Information, Monosodium Glutamate (MSG)."

FDA practice has been to name monosodium glutamate in the FDA's list of safe food ingredients:

FEDERAL FOOD, DRUG, AND COSMETICS ACT
Title 21 – Food and Drugs

Chapter 1 – Food and Drug Administration Department of Health and Human Services

SUBCHAPTER B — FOOD FOR HUMAN CONSUMPTION

Part 182 – Substances generally recognized as safe

Subpart A—General provisions

Sec. 182.1 Substances that are generally recognized as safe

(a) It is impracticable to list all substances that are generally recognized as safe for their intended use. However, by way of illustration, the Commissioner regards such common food ingredients as salt, pepper, vinegar, baking powder, and monosodium glutamate as safe for their intended use.

In the January-February 2003 *FDA Consumer* magazine, Michelle Meadows spewed out paragraphs that look like they came right off the Web pages of The Glutamate Association and the International Glutamate Information Service, which gave the appearance of trying to convince consumers that processed free glutamic acid is "safe" while saying nothing of merit. The article was titled, "MSG: A Common Flavor Enhancer."

In the late 1980s, the FDA established an Adverse Reactions Monitoring system (ARMS) concerned with the retrieval, processing, and analysis of data related to adverse health effects associated with specific food products and additives. The ARMS was a passive surveillance system allegedly designed to identify specific areas for focused clinical investigations on potentially causal associations. At one time, ARMS collected (not solicited, just collected) reports of adverse reactions to aspartame, monosodium glutamate, and sulfites. But in 1998 when a lawsuit demanding full labeling of MSG was dropped, the FDA stopped accepting reports of adverse reactions following ingestion of MSG or aspartame (the two excitotoxic amino acids used in food).

When called upon to investigate charges that the behavior of the FDA was inappropriate, the FDA/HHS Office of the Inspector General made sure that the investigation would be killed by turning it over to the Office of Research Integrity, which under no circumstances would have jurisdiction in this matter.

When challenged in a lawsuit over full and clear labeling of MSG (August 29, 1995), the court considered nothing but the Administrative Record presented by the FDA. Studies that demonstrated MSG had toxic potential were not allowed as evidence because they were not submitted to the court by the FDA as part of its Administrative Record. The Administrative record was made up of material that the FDA needed in order to win its case (refusal to label MSG), plus a smattering of material from the opposition that had no bite to it, but to which the FDA could point and say, "we looked at that."

The FDA has distorted results of its own research to serve the propaganda needs of the glutamate industry. In a 1995 study, the FDA's D.H. Daniels, F.L. Joe, and G.W. Diachenko misrepresented their own data about the toxicity of monosodium glutamate, also misrepresenting research findings of others (1).

In 1971, the FDA's J.F. Lynch, L.M. Lewis, and J.S. Adkins reported that hyperglycemia along with growth suppression followed ingestion of MSG and noted that hyperglycemia did not occur when subjects were given intact protein containing a large amount of glutamate – an observation that the FDA has chosen to ignore in favor of promoting the glutamate industry line that the L-glutamate in monosodium glutamate and in the human body are identical in all ways (2).

Historically, in setting up reviews of the safety (never toxicity) of monosodium glutamate, the FDA has contracted with groups that provided consultants with strong ties to the glutamate industry, and/or structured their allegedly "independent" reviews to consider only industry-approved data.

Historically, every time concern about MSG toxicity has intensified, the FDA has called for an "independent" review of the safety of MSG and has, thereby, stalled addressing the issue of MSG toxicity.

In 1992, the FDA contracted with FASEB to do an "independent" review of the safety of MSG in food. Every aspect of that study was marked by lack of objectivity and FDA/FASEB pro-industry bias. In its Request for Proposal, for example, the FDA asked questions that could not be answered, appointed Expert Panel members (at least four of the eight members selected by FASEB) who had ties to the glutamate industry, and attempted to eliminate relevant non-industry-produced data from consideration.

Legislators who inquired about the safety of MSG at that time were routinely told that the issue was being studied.

Manufacturers who inquired about the safety of MSG were told there was a study under way.

When a draft of the FASEB final report was submitted to the FDA in September 1994, that top-secret report was shared with the glutamate industry, found unacceptable, and sent back to FASEB by the FDA for "further study" — with instructions that FASEB should include the misinformation that consumers would not react to less than 2.5 or 3 grams of processed free glutamic acid taken in a single meal. This was the path designed to pave the way for calling for a labeling threshold of 3.0 grams or more processed free glutamic acid (but not less than 3.0 grams processed free glutamic acid) if in the future the glutamate industry considered it necessary to allege that all MSG in processed food was identified through food labeling.

The FDA/FASEB contract to provide "clarification" was signed February 1, 1995. The new contract provided the FDA with ammunition that they would use for refusing to identify all MSG in processed food if, in the future, they might be pressured to do so.

Everything about that contract and the way in which it was executed suggests that the FDA/FASEB report published in 1995 was undertaken in order to justify the FDA's refusal to require that all MSG in processed food be labeled.

Specifically, the FDA asked FASEB to review data relevant to possible limitations on the use of glutamates and to review data relevant to recommendations for special labeling requirements, and/or recommended levels of use of glutamates. As if to guarantee the outcome of the FASEB report, the FDA, in the "Background Section" of its contract, referred to evidence that people react to doses of 3 grams or more of MSG, but failed to refer to evidence (from the same study as well as others) that people react to doses of less than 3 grams of MSG. The FDA also mentioned, in its new contract, that asthma can be "worsened" with doses of more than 2.5 grams of MSG, but failed to mention that asthma can also be "worsened" with doses of less than 2.5 grams of MSG, and that MSG can trigger asthma-type attacks in non-asthmatics. Finally, the FASEB study's outcome was guaranteed by the facts that FASEB was required 1) to respond directly to questions asked by the FDA; 2) to respond only to questions asked by the FDA; and 3) to review certain data, while ignoring certain other data.

The FDA's rejection of the FASEB September 1994 draft final report on the safety of MSG in food was not without precedent. When FASEB submitted a report on the safety of MSG to the FDA in July 1978, the FDA returned the report "for updating in light of new information on these substances presented at an international symposium in May, 1978." The symposium in question had been sponsored by the glutamate industry, and, with rare exception, the research reported had been sponsored by it as well.

Following the 1995 release of the "independent" FASEB report, the FDA published an Advance Notice of Proposed Rulemaking which reinforced the design for labeling some processed free glutamic acid, but not all processed free glutamic acid, if the FDA was forced to label processed free glutamic acid. The point was to set the minimum for labeling at 3.0 grams of processed free glutamic acid which would ensure that some, but not all, processed free glutamic acid would be labeled and that most would remain unlabeled. This was notice of a possible proposal, not an actual proposal on which the public could formally comment.

Controlling reviews of the "safety" (never "toxicity") of MSG has not been the glutamate industry's only strategy for proving that monosodium glutamate is a harmless food additive.

Their power can be seen in the FDA's appointment of Andrew G. Ebert, Ph.D., then chairman of the IGTC, and Kristen McNutt, Ph.D., J.D., a spokesperson sponsored by The Glutamate Association, to the FDA Food Advisory Committee — and the FDA's refusal to appoint a single person who might be considered a legitimate consumer advocate.

The appointment of McNutt and Ebert, and refusal to appoint a true consumer advocate, demonstrate a clear-cut conflict of interest. Ebert's appointment, and the subsequent refusal to dismiss him, also demonstrate the FDA's complicity in blatant scientific fraud.

Why fraud? Because Ebert had distributed both test materials and material that he called placebos (allegedly inert substances that could not possibly cause a physical reaction in a person who ingested them) for use in double-blind studies designed to demonstrate that monosodium glutamate is safe. And the supposed placebos that Ebert distributed were not inert substances at all, but, known to Ebert, contained aspartame, a substance made up of aspartic acid, phenylalanine, and a methyl esther. Aspartic acid is a neurotoxic amino acid and structural analog of glutamic acid, the neurotoxic ingredient in MSG. Both aspartic acid and glutamic acid cause brain lesions, retinal deterioration, and neuroendocrine disorders in laboratory animals. In addition, the adverse reactions to aspartame on file with the FDA are literally the same reactions reported to the FDA by people who are sensitive to MSG. Even the relative frequencies with which the reactions occur are the same. Could it be by other than purposeful intent that Ebert not only compromised the integrity of the placebo, but used in his placebos a substance that would not only guarantee adverse reactions in people who were exposed to amounts that exceeded their dose tolerance levels, but would precipitate the same reactions as monosodium glutamate?

THE FACE AT THE FDA

Michael Taylor was industry's man at the FDA for a number of years, serving as the Deputy Commissioner there from 2010 to 2016. He came from Monsanto, producer of Glyphosate, Roundup's active ingredient and the most widely used herbicide in the United States, and leader in creation and sales of genetically modified organisms (GMOs).

To our knowledge, Taylor has never worked directly for Ajinomoto. But Ajinomoto and Monsanto have worked closely together for years. And Taylor was there front and center on *60 Minutes* for the glutamate industry when the glutamate industry was looking for someone to testify to the safety of monosodium glutamate. Who better to testify to the safety of monosodium glutamate on CBS than someone at the FDA?

Until it was made public that Ajinomoto's agent in charge of research was supplying his researchers with placebos that would cause the same reactions as those caused by MSG, Andrew Ebert, Ph.D., Chairman of Ajinomoto's International Glutamate Technical Committee was Ajinomoto's agent in charge of research.

THE BIG PICTURE

You have to understand just how the game is played in order to appreciate the hold that industry has on every branch of government in this country, on a large part of the scientific community, and on the media. If MSG was ever identified on food labels, consumers might notice that MSG was possibly causing or exacerbating illness and disease and exposing that fact would cost the glutamate industry billions of dollars in lost revenues. So researchers are hired to turn out research that claims to have demonstrated the safety of MSG; physicians, "scientists," and public relations firms are hired to fabricate stories about the safety of MSG; and the FDA, and the U.S. Department of Agriculture (USDA), and the Environmental Protection Agency (EPA) do the bidding of the rich and powerful food, drug, and cosmetic industries — declaring that their toxic products are "safe." And the people we have elected to public office ignore the fact that millions of pounds of neurotoxic MSG are being fed to our children, ourselves, and the elderly, that millions of people are suffering because of it and that the use of this excitotoxic amino acid in processed food contributes exponentially to the cost of health care in this country.

It's the same game that is currently being played by Ajinomoto over its aspartame interests and by Monsanto/Bayer over Roundup, glyphosate, and GMOs. It's the same game that was played for years by the cigarette industry.

The FDA is diametrically opposed to informing consumers about where MSG is hidden in food. For two decades, the glutamate industry, led by Ajinomoto Company, Inc. and the FDA, and the USDA maintained that MSG did not cause or exacerbate brain lesions or neuroendocrine disorders. Later, no longer able to deny the relationship between MSG and brain lesions, the glutamate industry, moved to the argument that brain lesions and neuroendocrine disorders can be caused by MSG, but only in laboratory animals, and that what applies to laboratory animals does not apply to humans. And the FDA and the USDA made no comment.

The animal studies were followed by carefully rigged human studies, none of which were questioned by the FDA. In fact, the FDA had approved the protocols for many of them. The question of glutamate-induced brain damage had been summarily dismissed by MSG's manufacturer, and the producers of ingredients that contained MfG (including MSG) only focused on convincing consumers and healthcare professionals that MfG wouldn't cause adverse reactions. There was no mention of brain damage.

To provide a fail-safe to guard against the possibility that down the road the House or Senate might insist on transparency in MSG labeling, the glutamate industry changed its strategy for assuring that MSG would not be honestly labeled. Instead of having the FDA claim that essentially no one is sensitive to MSG, Ajinomoto and friends would agree to labeling some MSG, but not all MSG. They would agree to labeling MSG only when found in amounts that far exceeded the amounts of MSG presently found in processed food.

And if you are concerned? You, the taxpayer? You, the voter? Industry depends on the fact that most consumers will throw up their hands in frustration and disgust and do nothing. Industry also depends on the fact that they control the media. Not since 1991 when 60 Minutes did its segment on MSG (which got national coverage), has there been a negative mention about MSG in any major media outlet.

When it was demonstrated to the FDA that all of the research that had been submitted as evidence that monosodium glutamate was a harmless food additive was flawed — flawed to the point of being fraudulent (3) — the FDA did nothing.

MSG is all about money. Both in and out of the FDA.

APPENDIX NOTES

1. Daniels, D.H., Joe, F.L. and Diachenko, G.W. (1995). Determination of free glutamic acid in a variety of foods by high-performance liquid chromatography. *Food Additives and Contaminants* 12:21-29.

2. Lynch, JF Jr, Lewis LM, Adkins JS. Monosodium glutamate-induced hyperglycemia in weanling rats. *Fed Proc.* 1971;30(2):460Abs (Abstract #1477).

3. The term 'fraud' is generally defined in the law as an intentional misrepresentation of material existing fact made by one person to another with knowledge of its falsity and for the purpose of inducing the other person to act, and upon which the other person relies with resulting injury or damage. [Fraud may also include an omission or intentional failure to state material facts, knowledge of which would be necessary to make other statements not misleading.] Accessed on 11/4/2010 at the 'Lectric Law Library's Lexicon.

About the Author

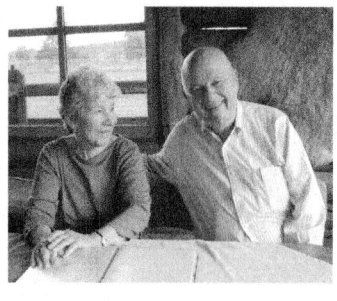

Adrienne Samuels, Ph.D., is co-founder and director of the Truth in Labeling Campaign, established in 1994 with her late husband, MSG activist Jack Samuels.

An experimental psychologist by training and educational psychologist by degree, she holds a B.S. degree from Northwestern University where she graduated with distinction and departmental honors. She received her Ph.D. from the University of Wisconsin, Madison where she studied with statisticians Chester Harris and Julian Stanley.

In 1988, in an attempt to better understand the etiology of Jack's life-threatening sensitivity to manufactured (man-made) free glutamic acid (MfG), Adrienne undertook an investigation of the literature on MSG's toxic reactions in animals and adverse reactions in humans, finding that MfG, the toxic component of MSG, is an excitotoxic (brain damaging) neurotoxin and endocrine disruptor, and that industry studies which claim otherwise are badly flawed.

She has shared her findings with the FDA and various members of Congress. She has testified before the Advisory Committee on the Food and Drug Administration and submitted testimony to the Federation of American Societies for Experimental Biology, Life Sciences Research Office, was a plaintiff in the lawsuit Truth in Labeling Campaign, et al., Plaintiffs vs. Donna Shalala, et al., Defendants (brought to require that MfG in processed food be identified on product labels), has filed

Citizen Petitions requesting that the FDA's GRAS (generally recognized as safe) status for MSG and MfG be withdrawn, and has filed Freedom of Information requests for (possibly non-existent) copies of studies on which the FDA has based those GRAS designations.

She currently maintains the Truth in Labeling Campaign websites, blogs, and social media pages for the benefit of MfG-sensitive people and others who choose to avoid the substance.

Adrienne's most recent focus has been on the well-concealed fact that MfG ingested in quantity by pregnant women will cause damage to the arcuate nucleus of the hypothalamus of the maturing fetus – the area of the brain that would have regulated appetite and satiety (weight control) had it not been obliterated by MfG. Drawing the distinction between the intractable obesity caused by glutamate-induced brain damage, and weight gain caused without brain damage, Adrienne has named this intractable condition "Type 2 Obesity."

Printed in Great Britain
by Amazon

36300526R00136